WORKBOOK FOR

OLDS' MATERNAL-NEWBORN NURSING & WOMEN'S HEALTH ACROSS THE LIFESPAN

WORKBOOK FOR

OLDS' MATERNAL-NEWBORN NURSING & WOMEN'S HEALTH ACROSS THE LIFESPAN

EIGHTH EDITION

MARCIA L. LONDON, RNC, MSN, APRN, CNS, NNP

*Senior Clinical Instructor and Director Neonatal Nurse Practitioner Program
Beth-El College of Nursing and Health Sciences at UCCS
University of Colorado of Colorado Springs, Colorado Springs, Colorado
Staff Clinical Nurse, Urgent Care
and After Hours Clinic, Colorado Springs, Colorado*

Patricia A. Wieland Ladewig, PhD, RN

*Professor and Academic Dean, School for Health Care Professions, Regis
University, Denver, Colorado*

Michele R. Davidson, PhD, CNM, CFN, RN

*Assistant Professor of Nursing and Women's Studies, George Mason
University, Fairfax, Virginia, Staff Nurse, Midwife, Women's Healthcare
Associates of Londoun, Lansdowne, Virginia*

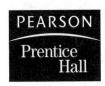

PEARSON
Prentice
Hall

Upper Saddle River, New Jersey

Publisher: Julie Levin Alexander
Assistant to Publisher: Regina Bruno
Editor-in-Chief: Maura Connor
Executive Acquisitions Editor: Pamela Lappies
Associate Editor: Michael Giacobbe
Development Editor: Alan Sorkowitz
Managing Editor, Development: Marilyn Meserve
Editorial Art Manager: Patrick Watson
Media Product Manager: John J. Jordan
Director of Marketing: Karen Allman
Senior Marketing Manager: Francisco del Castillo
Marketing Coordinator: Michael Sirinides
Managing Editor, Production: Patrick Walsh
Production Editor: Heather Willison, Carlisle
Production Liaison: Anne Garcia
Media Project Manager: Stephen Hartner
Manufacturing Manager: Ilene Sanford
Manufacturing Buyer: Pat Brown
Senior Design Coordinator: Maria Guglielmo
Printer/Binder: RR Donnelley, Willard
Composition: Carlisle Publishing Services
Cover Design: Cheryl Asherman
Cover Illustration: *Kaleidoscope VIII: The Sun, the Moon . . . and the Stars.*
A quilt designed and made by Paula Nadelstern, copyright 1991
Cover Printer: Phoenix Color

Pearson Education LTD.
Pearson Education Singapore, Pte. Ltd
Pearson Education, Canada, Ltd
Pearson Education–Japan
Pearson Education Australia PTY, Limited

Pearson Education North Asia Ltd
Pearson Educación de Mexico, S.A. de C.V.
Pearson Education Malaysia, Pte. Ltd
Pearson Education, Inc., Upper Saddle River, New Jersey

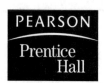

10 9 8 7 6 5 4 3 2 1
ISBN-13: 978-0-13-240149-4
ISBN: 0-13-240149-5

We dedicate this book to our families—with love.
David, Craig, and Matthew London
Tim, Ryan, and his wife, Amanda, and Erik Ladewig
Nathan, Hayden, Chloe, Caroline, and Grant Davidson

PREFACE

Maternal-newborn nurses are responsible for a complex, specialized body of knowledge related to the needs of the childbearing family, whether normal or at-risk. In recent years, that body of knowledge has expanded rapidly, as have the technologic and complex ethical issues surrounding pregnancy and birth. In addition, this knowledge base must be taught in a shorter period of time.

The *Olds' Maternal-Newborn Nursing & Women's Health Across the Lifespan Workbook* can assist in that effort by providing a concise, up-to-date review of maternal-newborn and women's health nursing care theoretical content, which emphasizes application of critical thinking in clinical and community-based maternity settings. Women's health issues are also explored.

All major maternity texts include content related to the human reproductive system and to the antepartal, intra-partal, postpartal, and neonatal periods, although the sequences of content may vary. This workbook can be used with most of the major maternity nursing texts, no matter what the organization. It is specifically designed to be used with *Olds' Maternal-Newborn Nursing & Women's Health Across the Lifespan,* Eighth Edition, by Davidson, London, and Ladewig. The subjects follow the same sequence as in the textbook, although a few textbook chapters are combined into one workbook chapter. To assist the student, we have identified the pertinent corresponding text chapters at the beginning of each workbook chapter and in the table of contents. MediaLinks to the Companion Website and Student DVD-ROM are identified on each chapter opening page. The workbook is appropriate for all types of nursing programs. Nurses involved in refresher courses or just entering this specialty area will also find it extremely helpful. Practicing nurses can find it helpful, too, especially in assessment and critical clinical decision making.

FEATURES OF THIS EDITION

By its very nature, maternal-newborn nursing is community-based nursing. Only a brief portion of the entire pregnancy and birth is spent in a birthing center or hospital. Moreover, because of changes in practice, even women with high-risk pregnancies are receiving more care in their homes and in the community and spending less time in hospital-based settings. The provision of nursing care in community-based settings is a driving force in health care today and, conse-quently, questions on community-based care are included throughout this workbook. Because we believe that sound clinical judgment develops from theoretic knowledge, research, and practical experience, most of the items in this workbook are based on clinical situations. Recognizing the rich cultural heritage of our diverse population, many of these client situations include ethnic families.

At the beginning of each chapter in this workbook, you will find a MediaLink box. Just as in the main textbook, this box identifies for you—the student—all the specific media resources and activities available for that chapter on the DVD-ROM, found in the main textbook, and Companion Website. You will find reference to video clips from the DVD-ROM, and case studies and care plans from the Companion Website to help you visualize and comprehend difficult concepts. Chapter by chapter, this MediaLink box hones your critical thinking skills and enables you to apply concepts from the book into practice.

This workbook also emphasizes the application and synthesis of an expanding evidence-based, maternal-newborn nursing clinical knowledge. Because students learn best through active learning, we have provided critical thinking scenarios to further develop critical decision-making and prioritizing skills. *Critical Thinking Challenge* situations are presented, and the student is asked to prioritize nursing actions. *Critical Thinking in Practice* sequences have been developed for selected normal and complication chapters to provide realistic clinical practice situations. Clinical data are presented, and the student is guided through the decision-making process for a particular situation.

Because of our strong belief in and years of working with students, we have *Nursing Care Plan in Action* scenarios. We have found that the variety of Care Pathway formats in clinical use may not be the most effective learning tool for student nurses preparing for clinical experience. Nursing Care Plans (NCPs) continue to be valued as a learning strategy and remain a mainstay in many nursing programs.

Working with the childbearing family is an intensely rewarding interactive nursing experience. The review of these clinical experiences and/or a personal childbearing experience increases our understanding of the universal childbirth/parenting experience. We have provided the student with opportunities in the *Reflections* feature. The purpose of this learning tool is to encourage the student to revisit and ponder these experiences, and in addition, to take full advantage of the journaling technique as a valuable method of learning.

Lastly, we have provided answers to all questions at the end of the book. Some of the questions are factual and can be verified in the textbook. Other questions require decision making or application of clinical judgment. The answers for these questions reflect our own experience, knowledge, and clinical practice.

CLARIFICATION OF TERMS

Although we recognize that the men in nursing are becoming more involved in the provision of maternity care, women are still the major care providers. Therefore, whenever possible, we have avoided gender-specific pronouns in referring to the nurse. When this was not possible, we have used the female pronoun.

By the same token, we appreciate the fact that the individual who is most significant to the pregnant woman may be her husband, the father of the child, another family member, or simply a good friend, male or female. Thus we have provided both traditional "husband-wife" situations, and situations involving other support persons.

ACKNOWLEDGMENTS

First, we would like to recognize the students who reviewed the previous edition of this workbook. They approached their review seriously and provided many candid comments. They identified material that they felt was unclear and added valuable suggestions that enhance this edition.

We thank the nurse educators and practicing nurses who reviewed this material and offered their suggestions and comments. Their input helped us focus on the most pertinent material and offered a broader perspective.

Last but not least, we thank our families. We recognize the countless ways that they continue to help us and the sacrifices that they make as we pursue this other love. Women can accomplish any goal; however, combining marriage, family, intellectual challenges, and a career requires a supportive, adaptive, responsive family. Each of us is blessed with such a family. We love them.

M.L.L.
P.W.L.
M.R.D.

CONTENTS

WORKBOOK FOR

OLDS' MATERNAL-NEWBORN NURSING & WOMEN'S HEALTH ACROSS THE LIFESPAN

CHAPTER 1

CONTEMPORARY MATERNAL-NEWBORN CARE

This chapter provides an introduction to some of the concepts that help shape maternal-newborn nursing and women's health care. It also briefly addresses concepts related to the care of the family in a culturally diverse society and concludes with basic information on complementary and alternative care. It corresponds to Chapters 1, 2, and 3 in the eighth edition of *Olds' Maternal-Newborn Nursing & Women's Health Across the Lifespan*.

CONTEMPORARY CHILDBIRTH

1. List at least three changes that have occurred in childbirth practices over the past 25 years.

   a.

   b.

   c.

NURSING ROLES

2. Maternity nurses function in a variety of roles in providing care to childbearing families. Define each of the following roles with emphasis on educational background and scope of function:

   a. Professional nurse

   b. Clinical nurse specialist (CNS)

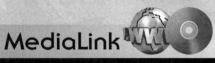

MediaLink

http://www.prenhall.com/davidson

Additional resources for this content can be found on the Student DVD-ROM accompanying the eighth edition of *Olds' Maternal-Newborn Nursing & Women's Health Across the Lifespan*, and on the Companion Website at http://www.prenhall.com/davidson. Click on the text chapter number(s) listed for this content to select the appropriate activities.

Prentice Hall Nursing MediaLink DVD-ROM
- Audio Glossary
- NCLEX Review
- Tools: Common Abbreviations in Maternal-Newborn Nursing

Companion Website
- Additional NCLEX Review
- Case Study: Cord Blood Banking
- Case Study: Family Assessment
- Case Study: Complementary Therapies
- Care Plan Activity: Midcycle Pain in Perimenopausal Women
- Care Plan Activity: Use of CAM in High-Risk Adolescent Pregnancy
- Tools: Common Abbreviations in Maternal-Newborn Nursing

   c. Nurse practitioner (NP)

   d. Certified nurse-midwife (CNM)

3. Which of the following would be most qualified to provide prenatal,
   intrapartal, postpartal, and newborn care for the low-risk
   childbearing woman?

   a. Acute care clinical nurse specialist

   b. Certified nurse-midwife

   c. Lay midwife

   d. Obstetric or women's healthcare nurse practitioner

COMMUNITY-BASED NURSING CARE

4. The three areas of focus of primary care include _____,
   _____, and _____.

5. Primary care is best provided in a _____ setting.

6. Identify two purposes of home care.

   a.

   b.

STANDARDS OF CARE

7. Discuss the standards of care that shape maternal-newborn nursing.

8. Identify four elements that must be addressed to ensure informed consent by a client.

   a.

   b.

   c.

   d.

REFLECTIONS

There are many difficult ethical issues affecting the childbearing woman and family today. What do you think the most difficult issue will be for you in your maternal-newborn nursing course?

_____

_____

_____

_____

_____

_____

9. The following descriptive statistics are one form of data that can be used to support evidence-based practice. Define each one.

   a. Birth rate

   b. Infant mortality rate

   c. Neonatal mortality rate

   d. Maternal mortality rate

10. Identify factors that might contribute to the decrease in the maternal mortality rate.

11. The perinatal mortality rate is a combination of the

    a. infant death rate and neonatal mortality rate.

    b. fetal death rate and infant death rate.

    c. neonatal mortality rate and postneonatal mortality rate.

    d. fetal death rate and neonatal mortality rate.

EVIDENCE-BASED NURSING PRACTICE

12. Briefly define *evidence-based practice*.

THE CONTEMPORARY FAMILY

13. Define *family*.

14. A family in which the parents are divorced and the children are members of two households, that of the father and that of the mother, is termed a/an

    a. binuclear family.

    b. blended family.

    c. extended family.

    d. kin network.

15. The beliefs, values, attitudes, and practices that are accepted by a population, a community, or an individual are termed _____.

16. Briefly describe ways in which a couple's religious beliefs might have an impact on their childbearing or childrearing practices.

COMPLEMENTARY AND ALTERNATIVE CARE

17. Compare *complementary* therapies and *alternative* therapies.

For the forms of complementary and alternative care in the following list, choose the appropriate definition from the column on the right.

18. _____ Acupuncture

19. _____ Alexander technique

20. _____ Ayurveda

21. _____ Biofeedback

22. _____ Feldenkreis

23. _____ Homeopathy

24. _____ Naturopathy

25. _____ Reflexology

26. _____ Reiki

a. Healing system that uses the concept of like to cure like

b. Form of therapy that uses the hands to transfer energy and restore balance

c. System of medicine based on the balance of energy or *chi*

d. Form of massage involving application of pressure to key points on hands, feet, or ears

e. Technique designed to help individuals learn to control their physiologic responses

f. Classic system of Hindu medicine aimed at helping people lead healthy lives

g. A movement-education technique based on proper alignment of head, neck, and trunk

h. System that uses a variety of natural approaches to preventing and treating problems

i. System based on concepts of movement reeducation

j. Technique that uses fine needles to stimulate pressure points

CHAPTER 2

WOMEN'S HEALTH CARE

Throughout her life a woman's healthcare needs change. In addition to age, these changing needs may be influenced by a variety of factors such as her family history, her plans for childbearing, her sexual activities, and any abnormal findings that develop. This chapter corresponds to Chapters 4 and 5 in the eighth edition of *Olds' Maternal-Newborn Nursing & Women's Health Across the Lifespan*.

COMMUNITY-BASED NURSING CARE

1. Summarize the concept of *women's health*.

THE ROLE OF THE NURSE IN MENSTRUAL COUNSELING

Match the definitions listed on the right with the correct terms in the following list.

2. _____ Amenorrhea	a.	Abnormally short menstrual cycle
3. _____ Hypomenorrhea	b.	Absence of menses
4. _____ Menorrhagia	c.	Excessive menstrual flow
5. _____ Dysmenorrhea	d.	Bleeding between periods
6. _____ Hypermenorrhea	e.	Painful menses
7. _____ Metrorrhagia	f.	Abnormally long menstrual cycle

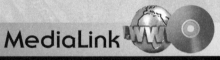

MediaLink

http://www.prenhall.com/davidson

Additional resources for this content can be found on the Student DVD-ROM accompanying the eighth edition of *Olds' Maternal-Newborn Nursing & Women's Health Across the Lifespan*, and on the Companion Website at http://www.prenhall.com/davidson. Click on the text chapter number(s) listed for this content to select the appropriate activities.

Prentice Hall Nursing MediaLink DVD-ROM
- Audio Glossary
- NCLEX Review

Companion Website
- Additional NCLEX Review
- Case Study: Premenstrual Girl
- Case Study: Family Planning
- Care Plan Activity: Bone Injuries in Postmenopausal Woman
- Care Plan Activity: Fertility Awareness
- Common Gynecologic Cancers

REFLECTIONS

Some women view menstruation as a normal, even welcome, part of life; some women view it as a minor annoyance; some women are embarrassed by it; others consider it a "curse" and hate it. Take a few moments to explore your views on menstruation. Try to identify some of the factors that have influenced your attitudes about it.

_____

_____

_____

_____

_____

_____

8. Discuss premenstrual syndrome (PMS) with regard to etiology, signs and symptoms, and treatment. Include information on self-care measures women with PMS might employ.

9. Identify five lifestyle choices a woman can make to improve her health and sense of well-being.

   a.

   b.

   c.

   d.

   e.

MENOPAUSE

10. Define *perimenopause.*

11. Perimenopause is characterized by (a) _____, (b) _____, and (c) _____.

12. Mrs. Joan Sanchez, age 50, has been coming to this office for her gynecologic exams for the past 7 years. Last year, she mentioned some irregularity in her periods. During her annual physical exam and Pap smear, she tells you that her periods have been more irregular and her last period was about 3 months ago. In addition, she has been experiencing difficulty sleeping; a sense of heat rising over her chest, neck, and face; increased perspiration; and palpitations. You identify that Mrs. Sanchez is entering menopause. In your counseling session, what information about self-care measures can you provide?

13. **Critical Thinking Challenge:** The following situation has been included to challenge your critical thinking. Read the situation and then answer the question "yes" or "no."

    Yvonne Swenson, age 52, is being seen for her annual examination. Her history reveals that she is a slender woman of Swedish ancestry who completed menopause at age 46. She does not drink alcohol but does smoke three fourths of a pack of cigarettes per day. She has two children.

    Is Ms. Swenson at increased risk of developing osteoporosis?

    Yes _____   No _____

    Explain your answer:

14. In women who have a uterus and who are on hormone replacement therapy (HRT), the estrogen is opposed by

    giving (a) _____ for all or part of the cycle to prevent the increased risk of

    developing (b) _____.

15. Which of the following is a risk factor for osteoporosis?

    a. African American race

    b. Lack of regular exercise

    c. Late onset of menopause

    d. Multiparity

CONTRACEPTIVE METHODS

For each of the following methods of contraception, select the appropriate mechanism of action from the list on the right.

16. _____ Condom

17. _____ Subdermal implants

18. _____ Diaphragm

19. _____ Depo-Provera

20. _____ Combined oral contraceptive

a. Prevents ovulation

b. Prevents transport of sperm to the ovum

21. When using a diaphragm, the woman should use additional spermicide before intercourse if more than

    (a) _____ hours have elapsed since the diaphragm was inserted. She should leave

    the diaphragm in place for at least (b) _____ hours after intercourse.

22. Marcella Heidegger has two children by a previous marriage. She has just begun seeing a man and asks you if the IUD would be a good contraceptive method if they become sexually involved. How would you respond?

23. The male sterilization procedure is called (a) _____; female sterilization is called

    (b) _____.

24. An estrogen-related side effect of oral contraceptives is

    a. acne.

    b. decreased libido.

    c. hirsutism.

    d. hypertension.

25. The contraceptive patch (Ortho Evra) provides (a) _____ hormonal protection. It is changed (b) _____ for 3 weeks, and then no patch is worn for (c) _____.

26. The NuvaRing vaginal contraceptive ring is left in place in the vagina for (a) _____ days. It is then removed for (b) _____ days.

27. What is the primary difference between the long-lasting injectable contraceptives, Lunelle and Depo-Provera?

    _____

    _____

28. Emergency postcoital contraception is indicated when a woman is concerned about the possibility of an unplanned pregnancy because of either (a) _____ or (b) _____. The emergency postcoital contraceptive must be started within (c) _____ hours of intercourse.

29. Medical abortion is possible during the first (a) _____ weeks of pregnancy. Once the length of pregnancy is confirmed, the woman takes a dose of (b) _____ in her caregiver's office. One to 3 days later she returns to the office to take a dose of (c) _____.

30. Warning signs that the woman may have developed a rare complication of the medical abortion regimen include (a) _____, (b) _____, (c) _____, and (d) _____.

31. What action should a woman take if she develops any of these signs?

CHAPTER 3

WOMEN'S HEALTH PROBLEMS

During her lifetime a woman may face a variety of health problems such as infections and gynecologic disorders. She is also at risk because of a myriad of social issues that pose a special challenge to women. This chapter considers those aspects of women's health care. It corresponds to Chapters 6, 7, 8, and 9 in the eighth edition of *Olds' Maternal-Newborn Nursing & Women's Health Across the Lifespan*.

COMMONLY OCCURRING INFECTIONS

Match the characteristic vaginal discharge listed on the right with the correct type of vaginitis.

1. _____ Bacterial vaginosis

2. _____ Trichomoniasis

3. _____ Vulvovaginal candidiasis

    a. Greenish white and frothy

    b. Thick, white, curdy

    c. Gray, milky

4. The presence of clue cells on a wet-mount preparation is indicative of

    a. bacterial vaginosis.

    b. chlamydia.

    c. trichomoniasis.

    d. vulvovaginal candidiasis.

For each of the following infections, select the appropriate antibiotic treatment from the list on the right for a woman who is not pregnant.

5. _____ Chlamydia

6. _____ Gonorrhea

7. _____ Syphilis

8. _____ Vulvovaginal candidiasis

    a. Benzathine penicillin G

    b. Butoconazole

    c. Ceftriaxone

    d. Azithromycin

9. **Critical Thinking in Practice:** The following action sequence is designed to help you think through clinical problems. Read the sequence, then fill in the appropriate boxes in the flowchart that follows.

Imagine you work as a registered nurse in a women's health clinic. It is your responsibility to interview women initially and obtain data on the purpose of their visits. You also do health teaching. You do not do pelvic examinations. Nita Singh, a client at the clinic, tells you she is there today because she has had marked itching of her vulva and vagina. She states, "It itches so bad that I've scratched it raw and made it worse." She tells you she has never had a vaginal infection before and has not been sexually active for 3 months. She says that she has had no symptoms of a urinary tract infection, although it does burn when the urine touches the excoriated skin.

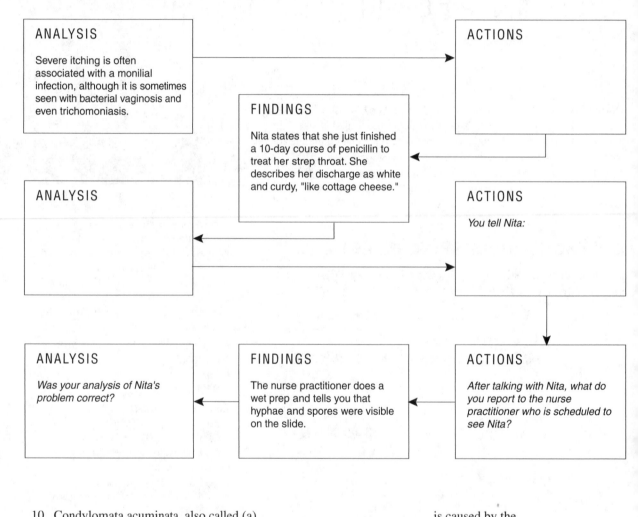

10. Condylomata acuminata, also called (a) _____, is caused by the

(b) _____. It is associated with an increased risk of (c) _____

_____.

11. The treatment of choice for pediculosis pubis is

a. acyclovir.

b. doxycycline.

c. metronidazole.

d. permethrin.

12. Mica Mihalko, diagnosed with trichomoniasis, has been given prescriptions for metronidazole for her and her partner. In addition to general teaching about the medication, what specific warning should you give Mica?

13. The greatest long-term problem caused by pelvic inflammatory disease (PID) is _____.

14. Compare cystitis and pyelonephritis.

	Cystitis	Pyelonephritis
Signs and symptoms		
Therapy		
Implications		
Client education		

DISORDERS OF THE BREAST

15. In performing a breast self-examination (BSE), why should a woman visually inspect her breasts with her arms in a variety of positions?

16. Explain the procedure for breast self-examination.

17. Which of the following findings during breast self-examination should a woman report to her healthcare provider?

    a. Difference in size between the breasts

    b. Silver-colored striae

    c. Symmetrical venous pattern

    d. Thickened skin with enlarged pores

Match the following conditions with the best description from the list on the right.

18. _____ Fibroadenoma

19. _____ Galactorrhea

20. _____ Duct ectasia

    a. Nipple discharge

    b. Excessive milk production in a lactating woman

    c. Tumor growing in the terminal portion of a breast duct

    d. Common, benign solid breast tumor

    e. Inflammation of the ducts behind the nipple

21. Your client experiences discomfort cyclically because of fibrocystic breast disease and asks if there are self-care measures she can use to alleviate her discomfort. What advice would you give her?

GYNECOLOGIC DISORDERS

22. The three most common symptoms of endometriosis are

    a. _____   b. _____   c. _____

23. In the office where you work as a nurse, one of the women being treated for endometriosis is going to begin taking danazol. You assess her knowledge level and find that she has only a vague understanding of the medication. Based on this assessment, what information would you give her about the drug?

24. A primary side effect of danazol (Danocrine) is

    a. dry, flaky skin.

    b. hirsutism.

    c. increased libido.

    d. weight loss.

25. Your client asks you about health practices she can follow to help her avoid developing toxic shock syndrome (TSS). What recommendations would you make?

Match the conditions listed with the most accurate definition from the column on the right.

26. _____ Lichen sclerosus   a. Inflammation of Bartholin's gland

27. _____ Vitiligo of the vulva   b. White, patchy areas of skin resulting from loss of pigmentation

28. _____ Vulvar vestibulitis   c. Benign condition characterized by white plaques and pruritus

                                               d. Inflammation and pain of the vulva at the vaginal entrance

29. When should women begin having Pap smears? _____

    _____

30. Anovulatory cycles with abnormal uterine bleeding that does not have a demonstrable organic cause is termed

    _____.

31. Downward displacement of the bladder into the vagina is termed (a) _____.

    Ballooning of the rectum into the vagina is called a (b) _____.

32. What do the initials TAH-BSO stand for? (a) _____. What is

    removed in the procedure? (b) _____

SOCIAL ISSUES

33. What two risk factors are most significant in predicting poverty in children?

    a.

    b.

34. Summarize the major components of the Personal Responsibility and Work Opportunity Reconciliation Act.

35. Discuss the impact of poverty on health care.

Environmental hazards in the workplace are often major concerns for women. Two agencies, OSHA and NIOSH, have been established to address the issue of environmental hazards in the workplace.

36. What does OSHA stand for? _____

37. What is the primary focus of OSHA?

38. What does NIOSH stand for? _____

39. What is the primary focus of NIOSH? _____

40. Elderly women are at increased risk of poverty. Identify at least four factors contributing to this problem.

   a.

   b.

   c.

   d.

41. Define *elder abuse.*

42. Identify the five types of elder abuse.

    a.

    b.

    c.

    d.

    e.

43. Identify four types of discrimination that lesbian and bisexual women may encounter.

    a.

    b.

    c.

    d.

VIOLENCE AGAINST WOMEN

44. Define *domestic violence.*

45. Estimates suggest that worldwide _____ in _____ women will be assaulted by a partner at some time in the woman's life.

46. Because female partner abuse is so common, many experts advocate universal screening of all female clients whenever they are seen by a healthcare provider. In caring for a nonpregnant woman, what are the three questions you should ask to screen for abuse?

    a.

    b.

    c.

47. You are caring for a woman who is abused, but she does not feel able to leave the situation. You encourage her to make an exit plan for herself and her children. What should be part of an exit plan?

Match the definitions on the right with the type of rape they best describe.

48. _____ Anger rape

49. _____ Confidence rape

50. _____ Power rape

51. _____ Sadistic rape

a. Assailant is known to the victim; previously the relationship was nonviolent

b. Assailant wishes to feel dominant and typically uses only the force necessary to subdue his victim

c. Attack is used to express feelings of rage and is often brutal and degrading

d. Planned assault characterized by torture, mutilation, and often murder

52. Briefly describe the Sexual Assault Nurse Examiner (SANE) Program.

CHAPTER 4

THE REPRODUCTIVE SYSTEM

Puberty represents a major milestone in a young person's life. Secondary sex characteristics develop, the reproductive organs mature, and the person becomes capable of procreation. This chapter reviews the female and male reproductive systems and the menstrual cycle, and reinforces the knowledge base from which maternity nursing care is derived.

This chapter corresponds to Chapter 10 in the eighth edition of *Olds' Maternal-Newborn Nursing & Women's Health Across the Lifespan*.

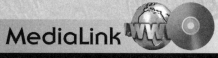

MediaLink

http://www.prenhall.com/davidson

Additional resources for this content can be found on the Student DVD-ROM accompanying the eighth edition of *Olds' Maternal-Newborn Nursing & Women's Health Across the Lifespan*, and on the Companion Website at http://www.prenhall.com/davidson. Click on the text chapter number(s) listed for this content to select the appropriate activities.

Prentice Hall Nursing MediaLink DVD-ROM
- Audio Glossary
- NCLEX Review
- Animation: 3-D Female Pelvis
- Activity: Female Reproductive System
- Activity: Ovulation
- Animation: 3-D Male Pelvis
- Activity: Male Reproductive System

Companion Website
- Additional NCLEX Review
- Case Study: Sex Education for Teens
- Care Plan Activity: Irregular Menses in a Client with Anxiety

FEMALE REPRODUCTIVE SYSTEM

Match the external genital structure with its function or characteristics during the childbearing period.

1. _____ Mons pubis

2. _____ Clitoris

3. _____ Labia minora

4. _____ Perineal body

5. _____ Paraurethral (Skene's) glands

6. _____ Vulvovaginal (Bartholin's) glands

a. Rich in sebaceous glands that lubricate and provide bactericidal secretions

b. Produces smegma that has a sexually stimulating odor

c. Protects pelvic bones, especially during coitus

d. Secretions lubricate vaginal vestibule to facilitate sexual intercourse

e. Secretes clear, thick mucus that enhances sperm viability and motility

f. Site of episiotomy and lacerations

PUBERTY

REFLECTIONS

Puberty comes as a surprise to some, whereas others are well prepared. How well prepared were you for the experience? What might you do or have you done to prepare your children for puberty? What are your memories of going through puberty?

_____

_____

_____

_____

7. Figure 4–1 shows the female internal reproductive organs. Identify the structures that are indicated.

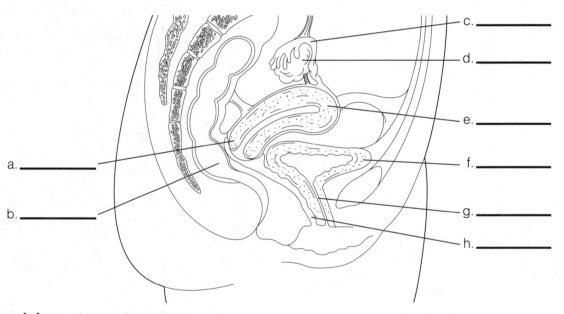

c. _____

d. _____

e. _____

a. _____

f. _____

b. _____

g. _____

h. _____

Figure 4–1   Female internal reproductive organs.

8. Briefly discuss the function(s) of the vagina.

9. What factors can alter the vagina's pH and decrease its self-cleansing action?

10. Label the uterine structures indicated in Figure 4–2.

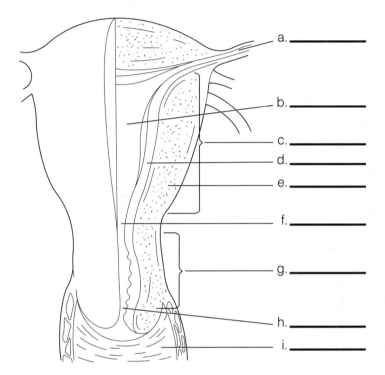

a. _____

b. _____

c. _____

d. _____

e. _____

f. _____

g. _____

h. _____

i. _____

Figure 4–2   Anatomy of the uterus.

11. The figure-eight pattern of the middle layer of uterine muscle fibers

    a. causes cervical effacement.

    b. constricts large uterine blood vessels when the fibers contract.

    c. forms sphincters at fallopian tube attachment sites.

    d. maintains the effects of uterine contractions during labor.

12. Briefly describe the function of the endometrium.

13. Identify three functions of the cervical mucosa.

    a.

    b.

    c.

14. A group of adolescents is waiting for pregnancy tests in a clinic. One of the girls asks about infections. The nurse explains that certain body functions protect the female from infection of the reproductive organs. Which of the following protects the female from infection of the reproductive organs?

    a. Alkaline pH and smegma secreted from the clitoris

    b. Acidic pH and bacteriostatic cervical mucosa

    c. Neutral pH of 7.5 and bactericidal secretions of the labia minora

    d. pH of 4 to 5 and secretions of the Skene's ducts

15. A nurse is teaching a class on the anatomy of the reproductive system. Which statement is correct regarding the function of the round ligament?

    a. It helps the fallopian tubes to "catch" the ovum each month.

    b. It keeps the uterus centrally placed in the pelvis.

    c. It contains sensory nerve fibers that contribute to dysmenorrhea.

    d. It steadies the uterus during labor and moves the fetus toward the cervix.

16. What are the primary functions of the fallopian tubes?

17. In relation to the fallopian tubes, what is the purpose or significance of each of the following?

    a. Fimbria

    b. Isthmus

    c. Ampulla

    d. Muscular layer

e. Nonciliated goblet cells of the mucosa

f. Tubal cilia

18. Briefly describe the function of the three layers (tunica albuginea, cortex, medulla) of the ovary.

19. What is (are) the primary function(s) of the ovaries?

20. Label the following pelvic bones and supporting ligaments in Figure 4–3.

Sacrum	Right sacroiliac joint	Sacrotuberous ligament
Left innominate bone	Sacroiliac ligament	Coccyx
Symphysis pubis	Sacrospinous ligament	

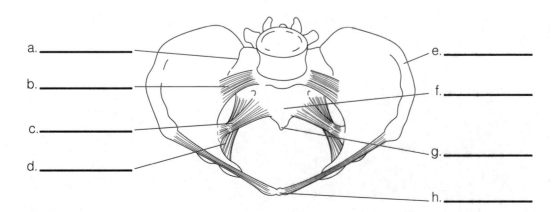

Figure 4–3   Bony pelvis with ligaments.

21. Figure 4–4 focuses on the muscles of the pelvic floor. Label the following structures:

Vagina   Iliococcygeus muscle   Pubococcygeus muscle
Bulbospongiosus muscle   Ischial tuberosity   External anal sphincter
Gluteus maximus muscle   Adductor longus muscle   Urogenital diaphragm
Ischiocavernosus muscle

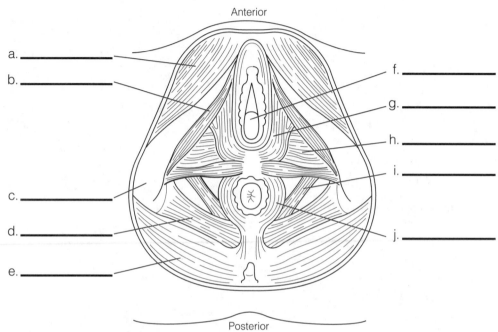

a. _____

b. _____

c. _____

d. _____

e. _____

f. _____

g. _____

h. _____

i. _____

j. _____

Anterior

Posterior

Figure 4–4   Muscles of the pelvic floor.

22. Define each of the following terms and briefly identify its implications for childbearing:

a. False pelvis

b. True pelvis

c. Pelvic inlet

d. Pelvic outlet

23. In Figure 4–5, label the false pelvis, true pelvis, pelvic inlet, and pelvic outlet.

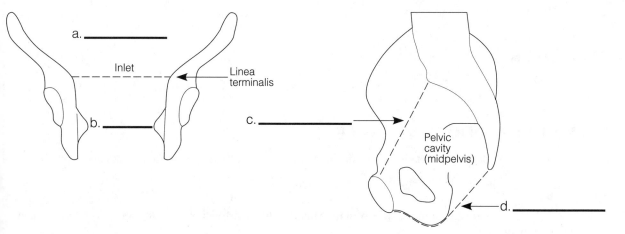

Figure 4–5 Pelvic divisions.

24. Label the major structures of the breast shown in Figure 4–6.

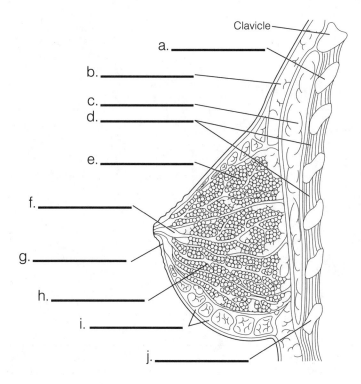

Figure 4–6 Anatomy of the breast shown in a sagittal section.

25. What is the primary function of the tubercles of Montgomery?

26. What portion of the breast contains the cuboidal epithelial cells that secrete the components of milk?

    a. Alveoli

    b. Ducts

    c. Lactiferous sinuses

    d. Lobules

FEMALE REPRODUCTIVE CYCLE

27. The female reproductive cycle (FRC) is made up of two interrelated cycles that occur simultaneously: the

    (a) _____ cycle and the (b) _____ cycle.

28. For each of the following hormones involved in ovulation and menstruation, state the source of secretion and the primary function(s).

Hormone	Source	Function(s)
Estrogen		
Progesterone		
Follicle-stimulating hormone (FSH)		
Luteinizing hormone (LH)		
Prostaglandins (PGE and PGF$_{2\alpha}$)		

29. A girl waiting for a pregnancy test asks the nurse which hormone causes ovulation to occur. The nurse explains that about 12 hours after the peak production of _____, ovulation occurs.

    a. estrogen

    b. FSH (follicle-stimulating hormone)

    c. LH (luteinizing hormone)

    d. progesterone

30. The nurse asks the girl to identify the hormone responsible for enhancing development of the graafian follicle and rebuilding the endometrium. The right answer would be

    a. estrogen.

    b. FSH–RH (follicle-stimulating hormone–releasing hormone).

    c. GnRH (gonadotropin-releasing hormone).

    d. LHRH (luteinizing hormone–releasing hormone).

31. Describe the process of ovulation and the related changes in the ovarian follicle.

32. Briefly describe the changes that occur in each of the following during the various phases of the menstrual cycle.

    a. Endometrium

    b. Cervical mucosa

33. Label the following components of the menstrual cycle in Figure 4–7, on page 28.

| Menstrual | Secretory | Follicular | Estrogen |
| Proliferative | Ischemic | Luteal | Progesterone |

MALE REPRODUCTIVE SYSTEM

34. The most important purpose for the location of the scrotum is to

    a. maintain temperature lower than that of the body.

    b. produce sperm near the point of ejaculation.

    c. protect the testes and sperm from the effects of the prostate.

    d. provide room for the convoluted seminiferous tubules.

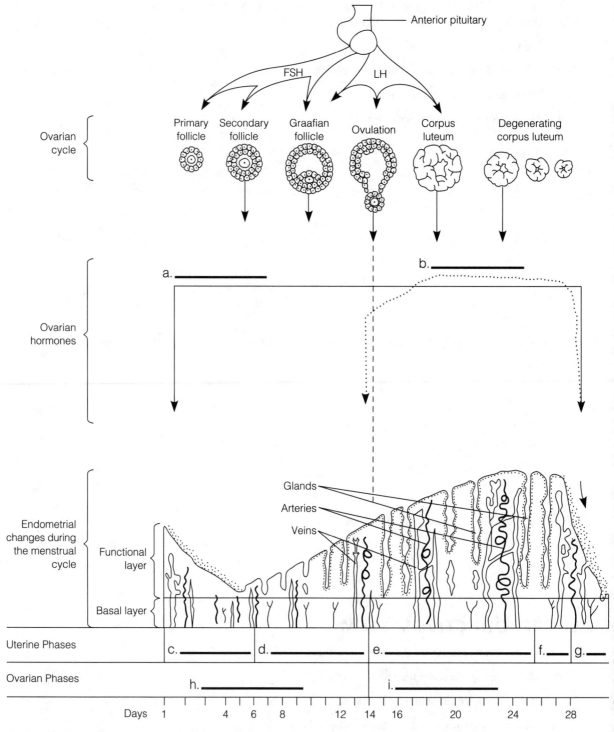

Figure 4–7 Female reproductive cycle: Interrelationships of hormones and the four phases of the uterine cycle and two phases of the ovarian cycle in an ideal 28-day cycle.

35. Complete the following sentences using the words related to the male reproductive structures and functions in the following list:

Bulbourethral (Cowper's) glands	penis	seminal vesicles
Epididymides	prostate gland	testis
ejaculatory duct	Sertoli's cells	testes
Leydig's cells	seminal fluid (semen)	vas deferens

The visible male reproductive organs include the (a) _____ and the scrotum. The

primary function of the scrotum is protection; it contains the (b) _____,

(c) _____, and (d) _____: the male internal reproductive structures.

Each (e) _____ produces testosterone via the (f) _____, and

houses the seminiferous tubules and immature sperm. Maturation of sperm occurs in the

(g) _____, the storage area for mature spermatozoa. Seminiferous tubules contain

(h) _____ cells, which nourish and protect the spermatocytes. The

(i) _____ secretes fluids high in fructose and prostaglandins that nourish sperm and

increase their motility. The vas deferens and the duct of a seminal vesicle unite to form a short tube called the

(j) _____, which passes through the prostate gland and terminates in the urethra. The

(k) _____ gland secretes thin, alkaline fluid containing calcium and other substances

that counteract the acidity of ductus and seminal vesicle secretions. The prostate gland secretes substances in

the (l) _____. The (m) _____ glands secrete viscous, alkaline

fluid rich in mucoproteins, which neutralize the acid in the male urethra and the vagina.

36. **Memory Check:** Define the following abbreviations.

a. FRC

b. FSH

c. GnRH

d. LH

Chapter 5

Conception, Fetal Development, and Special Reproductive Issues: Infertility and Genetics

The conception and development of a new human being is a never-ending source of awe and fascination.

This chapter begins with a review of the process of conception, implantation, placental functioning, and fetal development. Factors that may influence fetal development are explored, with special emphasis on the impact of maternal medications. Also discussed are the issues of infertility and the impact of genetics on reproduction. Most couples who want children are able to have them with little difficulty. In some instances, because of special reproductive issues, couples may be unable to fulfill their dream of having a baby.

This chapter corresponds to Chapters 11 and 12 in the eighth edition of *Olds' Maternal-Newborn Nursing & Women's Health Across the Lifespan.*

CELLULAR DIVISION

1. Briefly compare the differences between mitosis and meiosis.

2. Each sperm and ovum has (a)_____ chromosomes. When sperm and ovum are united, the resulting normal newborn has (b)_____ chromosomes.

3. The optimal time for fertilization to occur is (a)_____ hours after ovulation of the ovum and (b)_____ hours after ejaculation.

MediaLink

http://www.prenhall.com/ davidson

Additional resources for this content can be found on the Student DVD-ROM accompanying the eighth edition of *Olds' Maternal-Newborn Nursing & Women's Health Across the Lifespan,* and on the Companion Website at http:// www.prenhall.com/davidson. Click on the text chapter number(s) listed for this content to select the appropriate activities.

Prentice Hall Nursing MediaLink DVD-ROM
- Audio Glossary
- NCLEX Review
- Animation: Oogenesis
- Animation: Oogenesis and Spermatogenesis
- Animation: Cell Division
- Animation: Conception
- Animation: Embryonic Heart Formation and Circulation
- Animation Tutorial: Fetal Circulation
- Animation: Formation of Placenta
- Activity: Oogenesis and Spermatogenesis
- Activity: Ovulation

Companion Website
- Additional NCLEX Review
- Case Study: Teaching About Pregnancy
- Case Study: Infertility
- Care Plan Activity: Client Fearful of Multiple Gestation
- Care Plan Activity: Infertile Couple

4. The nurse explains capacitation and acrosomal reaction processes to a client in the fertility clinic. Which statement by the client indicates the nurse's explanation of capacitation was effective?

    a. Decreased motility of sperm is a characteristic of capacitation.

    b. Capacitation occurs in the male reproductive tract.

    c. Capacitation takes about 7 hours to complete.

    d. Decreased acrosomal reaction increases capacitation.

5. Fertilization occurs in the

    a. cervix.

    b. fallopian tube.

    c. ovary.

    d. uterus.

6. Briefly describe the process of fertilization.

7. The (a)_____ chromosome determines the sex of the child. The (b)_____ carries this chromosome.

8. A client tells you that her mother was a twin, two of her sisters have twins, and several cousins either are twins or gave birth to twins. The client is also expecting twins. Because there is a genetic predisposition to twinning in her family, there is a good chance that the client will have

    a. dizygotic twins.

    b. identical twins.

    c. monozygotic twins.

    d. nonzygotic twins.

CELLULAR MULTIPLICATION AND IMPLANTATION

The zygote continually develops as it travels through the fallopian tube to its site of implantation in the uterus. Match each of the following terms with the appropriate description.

9. _____ Cleavage   a. Period of rapid cellular division

10. _____ Blastomeres   b. Outer layer of cells that replaces the zona pellucida

11. _____ Morula   c. Small developing mass of cells held together by zona pellucida

12. _____ Blastocyst   d. Solid ball of cells

13. _____ Trophoblast   e. Inner solid mass of cells after cavity has formed

14. Implantation occurs about (a)_____ to (b)_____ days after fertilization. Briefly describe how implantation occurs.

15. After implantation, the portion of the endometrium that overlies the developing ovum is called

   a. decidua basalis.

   b. decidua capsularis.

   c. decidua luteum.

   d. decidua vera.

16. The mesoderm germ layer gives rise to the following structures:

   a. Alimentary canal, lungs, liver, and bladder

   b. Circulatory system, skin epithelium, and reproductive organs

   c. Muscles, lungs, and circulatory system

   d. Nervous system, lungs, and genitourinary system

EMBRYONIC MEMBRANES/AMNIOTIC FLUID/UMBILICAL CORD

17. The embryonic membranes begin to form at the time of implantation. Two distinct membranes develop: the

   (a)_____ and the (b)_____.

18. Using the terms from question 15 and your answers to question 17, fill in the blanks in Figure 5–1.

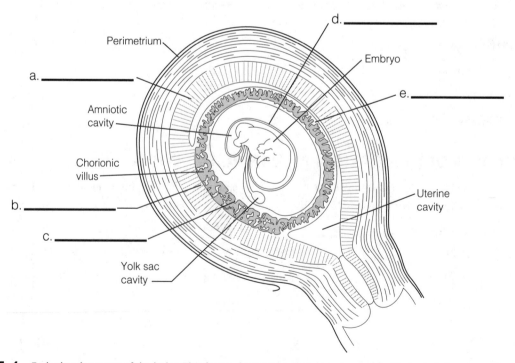

Figure 5–1 Early development of the baby. This figure depicts the early development of selected structures at approximately 8 weeks.

19. A nurse is teaching a prenatal group about amniotic fluid. Which statement by one of the group members indicates an understanding of factors associated with amniotic fluid volume? (Select all that apply.)

    a. About 600 mL amniotic fluid is swallowed by the fetus each day.

    b. About 400 mL of amniotic fluid flows out the fetal lungs every day.

    c. To prevent harm, the amniotic fluid restricts fetal movement.

    d. The fetus contributes to the volume of amniotic fluid by excreting urine.

20. When presenting information about fetal development to a group of high school girls, one of the girls asks the nurse to explain the functions of the amniotic fluid. The nurse's response should be, "The amniotic fluid cushions the embryo/fetus against mechanical injury, controls the embryo's temperature, and

    a. provides a means of nutrient exchange for the embryo/fetus."

    b. creates adherence of the amnion."

    c. allows freedom of movement so the embryo/fetus can change position."

    d. provides for fetal respiration and metabolism."

21. The body stalk, which attaches the embryo to the yolk sac, will develop into the umbilical cord. The umbilical cord is made up of (a)_____ vein(s), (b)_____ artery(ies), and specialized connective tissue called (c)_____, whose function is to (d)_____.

PLACENTA DEVELOPMENT AND FUNCTION

22. Describe the appearance of and the structures that make up the maternal and fetal side of the placenta.

23. List the four major placental hormones and their function during pregnancy.

Hormone	Function
a.	
b.	
c.	
d.	

24. Identify three major functions of the placenta.

    a.

    b.

    c.

25. Describe the visual assessments you would want to make of the placenta after birth.

26. Describe the following stages of human development in utero:

    a. Embryo

    b. Fetus

FETAL CIRCULATION

27. Circle the answer that correctly completes these sentences.

    The umbilical vein carries (**oxygenated**) or (**deoxygenated**) blood (**to**) or (**away from**) the fetus.

    The umbilical arteries carry (**oxygenated**) or (**deoxygenated**) blood (**from**) or (**to**) the fetus to the placenta.

28. Label the following structures in Figure 5–2 and, using arrows, trace the normal pathway of fetal circulation:

Umbilical vein   Ductus venosus   Inferior vena cava

Foramen ovale   Ductus arteriosus   Umbilical arteries

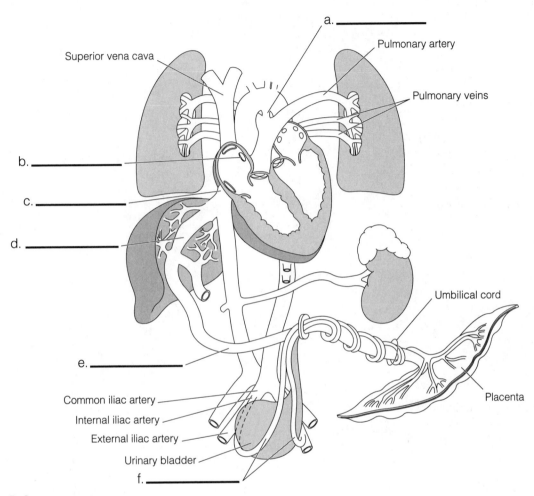

Figure 5–2   Fetal circulation.

29. Describe the function of each of the following fetal structures during fetal life and the changes that occur after birth in the newborn. (See Chapter 28 of text.)

	Fetal	Newborn
a. Umbilical vein		
b. Ductus venosus		
c. Inferior vena cava		
d. Foramen ovale		
e. Ductus arteriosus		
f. Umbilical arteries		

FETAL DEVELOPMENT

30. A fetus weighing about 780 g, measuring 28 cm in length, and who can make respiratory movements is approximately how many weeks' gestation?

    a. 14 weeks

    b. 18 weeks

    c. 20 weeks

    d. 24 weeks

31. You are assisting in a prenatal class on fetal development. Mrs. Elizabeth Oliver, a 22-year-old primigravida, is 14 weeks pregnant and has the following questions. Based on your knowledge of fetal development, how would you respond?

    a. "When will my baby look like a baby?"

    b. "How long is my baby now and how much does my baby weigh?"

    c. "When will I feel my baby move?"

    d. "When will my baby's heart start beating?"

    e. "When can my baby's sex be identified?"

    f. "Can my baby open its eyes?"

32. Identify three factors that influence embryonic and fetal development.

    a.

    b.

    c.

33. A nurse is teaching a class on healthy lifestyles during pregnancy. The teaching plan for a client in the first trimester of pregnancy should include (Select all that apply.)

    a. the avoidance of hot tubs.

    b. the use of vitamins and folic acid before conception.

    c. the use of fat-soluble vitamins E and K.

    d. the avoidance of glucose and fatty acids.

INFERTILITY

34. Define the following terms:

    a. Infertility

    b. Subfertility

REFLECTIONS

Feeling movement brings images of the future baby to moms and dads. What have parents told you about this, or what have you personally experienced?

_____

_____

_____

_____

_____

_____

_____

_____

_____

35. During a routine annual examination, your client tells you that she and her husband have been trying to conceive a child for about 8 months but have been unsuccessful. She asks you if there are any actions they can take to increase her chances of getting pregnant. What information would you give her?

36. Describe the correct procedure for taking the basal body temperature (BBT) and the changes in BBT that will occur throughout a woman's cycle if she is ovulating.

Match the following tests with their correct procedure or purpose.

37. _____ Cervical mucus tests (ferning, spinnbarkheit)

38. _____ Endometrial biopsy

39. _____ Postcoital test (Huhner test)

40. _____ Hysterosalpingography

41. _____ Gonadotropin levels (LH, FSH assays)

42. _____ Progesterone assay

43. _____ Transvaginal ultrasound

a. Detects changes in cervical mucus due to changing estrogen levels

b. Examination of uterine cavity and tubes using contrast media instilled through the cervix

c. Examination of cervical mucus for sperm motility

d. Examination of uterine lining for secretory changes and receptivity to implantation.

e. Detects ovulation and corpus luteum function

f. Detects follicular development and ovulatory function

g. Monitors developing follicle

44. Discuss semen analysis as a diagnostic tool in an infertility work-up. How is the semen collected? What findings indicate a normal semen analysis?

45. A male client is having a sperm analysis. The client states that he smokes one pack of cigarettes per day, exercises regularly, and follows a vegetarian diet plan. Which lab finding most likely would be based on this information collected by the nurse?

a. A decrease in sperm motility.

b. A decrease in sperm count.

c. A sperm pH level of 7.

d. A sperm count greater than 20 million/mL.

46. A nurse is teaching a client with infertility about the medication Clomid (clomiphene citrate). Which instructions should the nurse include in the teaching? (Select all that apply.)

    a. Avoid bright lighting when visual disturbances occur.

    b. Confirm the outcome with either a home pregnancy test or a serum blood test.

    c. Eight percent of women taking Clomid develop multiple-gestation pregnancies.

    d. Before injection, reconstitute the medication with a diluent.

47. For each of the following medications used to treat infertility, summarize the purpose, method of administration, and possible side effects:

    a. Human menopausal gonadotropin (Pergonal)

    b. Bromocriptine (Parlodel)

48. Victor Priolo's father has Huntington disease and Victor is exhibiting mild symptoms of the disorder. In order to eliminate any possibility of transmitting the disease to their offspring, Victor and his wife Ann are considering therapeutic insemination. An effective procedure would be to use

    a. donor sperm, implanted in Ann.

    b. Victor's sperm, implanted in a surrogate mother.

    c. Victor's sperm, implanted in Ann after genetic restructuring.

    d. donor sperm, implanted in Victor's sterilized testes.

49. Briefly describe the following reproductive technologies:

    a. Therapeutic insemination

    b. In vitro fertilization (IVF)

    c. Gamete intrafallopian transfer (GIFT)

    d. Tubal embryo transfer (TET)

    e. Micromanipulation and preimplantation genetic diagnosis (PGD)

50. As a nurse working in an office that focuses on infertility evaluation and treatment, it is your responsibility to coordinate care for couples, provide ongoing information and teaching, and evaluate the couple's psychosocial status. Dorothy Lewis, age 37, has had extensive testing and treatment in an effort to correct her infertility, but all approaches have failed. During a conversation with you, Dorothy expresses the feeling that she is a failure as a woman and a wife. She states, "We both think that children are an important part of marriage, but because of me, because my body can't do what it should, we are the losers. I am such a failure as a woman." Based on this information, formulate a possible nursing diagnosis that might apply, *and* identify some of the defining characteristics that led you to this diagnosis.

51. For infertile couples, the most difficult aspect of their problem is likely to be the

    a. decision to adopt or remain childless.

    b. emotional aspect.

    c. financial burden.

    d. painful and time-consuming testing.

GENETIC DISORDERS

52. The pictorial analysis of an individual's chromosomes is called a_____.

53. Your client's husband, who was adopted as an infant, has just been diagnosed as having Huntington chorea. Your client asks you what the possibility is that their two children will develop the disease. What is the correct answer? Diagram the pattern of inheritance, demonstrating your rationale for your response.

54. Tammy Daniel has cystic fibrosis. Because this is a condition of autosomal recessive inheritance, the nurse knows Tammy most likely inherited the disease from

    a. her father.

    b. her mother.

    c. both parents, who are carriers of the abnormal gene.

    d. neither parent, but as a result of a toxic environment in utero.

55. Identify the genetic problems that certain ethnic or age groups may be at risk for developing.

56. Draw a family tree (pedigree) for your family as far back as your grandparents, if possible. Are there any conditions your family considers hereditary? Don't forget to include findings such as high blood pressure, obesity, and diabetes. If you are not familiar with drawing family trees (pedigrees), you may find it helpful to consult a physical assessment text.

57. **Memory Check:** Define the following abbreviations.

    a. AF   d. hCS

    b. BBT   e. hMG

    c. hCG   f. hPL

CHAPTER 6

PHYSICAL AND PSYCHOLOGIC CHANGES OF PREGNANCY

As pregnancy progresses, a woman's body undergoes a variety of changes designed to support the growth and development of the fetus she is carrying. In addition to physical changes, the woman and her loved ones face major psychologic changes and adjustments. Life will never be the same. This chapter focuses on preparation for pregnancy and childbirth and the physical and psychologic changes that occur during pregnancy. It corresponds to Chapters 13 and 14 in the eighth edition of *Olds' Maternal-Newborn Nursing & Women's Health Across the Lifespan.*

PREPARATION FOR PREGNANCY AND CHILDBIRTH

1. Gretta Heidegger, a healthy 24-year-old woman, tells you that she and her partner are planning to begin their family soon. She asks what she should do during the preconception period to help ensure that she has a successful pregnancy. What would you tell her?

2. Define a *birth plan*.

MediaLink

http://www.prenhall.com/davidson

Additional resources for this content can be found on the Student DVD-ROM accompanying the eighth edition of *Olds' Maternal-Newborn Nursing & Women's Health Across the Lifespan* and on the Companion Website at http://www.prenhall.com/davidson. Click on the text chapter number(s) listed for this content to select the appropriate activities.

Prentice Hall Nursing MediaLink DVD-ROM
- Audio Glossary
- NCLEX Review

Companion Website
- Additional NCLEX Review
- Case Study: Preparing for Pregnancy
- Case Study: Prenatal Education
- Care Plan Activity: Preconception
- Counseling
- Care Plan Activity: Preparing Parents and Siblings for New Baby

3. During pregnancy, the expectant woman and her family begin to plan for their childbirth experience. Identify at least six issues a family should consider in their decision making.

   a.

   b.

   c.

   d.

   e.

   f.

4. With regard to philosophy and basic approaches, compare the psychoprophylactic (Lamaze) method of childbirth preparation to a method commonly used in your area.

ANATOMY AND PHYSIOLOGY OF PREGNANCY

5. The primary cause of uterine enlargement during pregnancy is the

   a. engorgement of preexisting vascular structures.

   b. formation of an additional layer of uterine musculature.

   c. hypertrophy of preexisting myometrial cells.

   d. increased number of myometrial cells.

6. How are the circulatory requirements of the uterus affected by pregnancy?

7. Many of the changes that occur in the pelvic organs during pregnancy are named. For each of the following changes, identify its correct name:

 a. The deep reddish purple coloration of the mucosa of the cervix, vagina, and vulva is called _____ sign.

 b. The softening of the cervix that occurs is called _____ sign.

 c. The softening of the isthmus of the uterus is called _____ sign.

8. During pregnancy, the increased number and activity of the endocervical glands are responsible for

 a. a marked softening of the cervix.

 b. a thinner, more watery mucosal discharge.

 c. the development of Chadwick's sign.

 d. the formation of the mucous plug.

9. What function does the mucous plug serve?

10. The ovaries _____ ovum production during pregnancy.

11. During the first 10 to 12 weeks of pregnancy, the corpus luteum

 a. gradually regresses and becomes obliterated.

 b. secretes estrogen to maintain the pregnancy.

 c. secretes human chorionic gonadotropin to maintain the pregnancy.

 d. secretes progesterone to maintain the pregnancy.

12. What is the significance of the increased acidity of the vaginal secretions during pregnancy?

13. Describe the breast changes that occur during pregnancy with regard to the following:

 a. Size

 b. Pigmentation

 c. Montgomery's tubercles

14. Why is there an increased tendency toward nasal stuffiness and epistaxis during pregnancy?

For the components of the cardiovascular system in the following list, indicate whether there is normally an increase (**I**) or a decrease (**D**) during pregnancy.

15. _____ Blood pressure

16. _____ Erythrocyte volume

17. _____ Cardiac output

18. _____ Hematocrit

19. _____ Pulse

20. The pseudoanemia of pregnancy is caused by

    a. a greater increase in plasma volume than in hemoglobin levels.

    b. decreased hemoglobin levels.

    c. a decrease in both plasma volume and hemoglobin levels.

    d. increased plasma volume without a comparable increase in hemoglobin levels.

21. During pregnancy, the enlarging uterus may cause pressure on the vena cava when the woman lies supine, interfering with returning blood flow. As a result the woman may feel dizzy and clammy, and her blood pressure may decrease. This condition is called the (a) _____ syndrome,

    (b) _____ compression, or (c) _____ syndrome.

22. Constipation during pregnancy is usually the result of

    a. prolonged stomach emptying time and decreased intestinal motility.

    b. increased peristalsis and flatulence.

    c. increased cardiac workload resulting in delayed peristalsis.

    d. reflux of acidic gastric contents and hypochlorhydria.

23. Identify the causes of each of the following discomforts of pregnancy:

    a. Heartburn

    b. Hemorrhoids

    c. Urinary frequency

24. Which of the following changes in kidney functioning occurs during a normal pregnancy?

    a. Blood urea nitrogen values increase.

    b. Glomerular filtration rate increases.

    c. Renal plasma flow decreases.

    d. Renal tubular reabsorption rate decreases.

Many changes occur in the skin during pregnancy. Match the terms identifying these changes with their appropriate definition from the column on the right:

25. _____ Chloasma (melasma)

26. _____ Striae gravidarum

27. _____ Spider nevi

28. _____ Linea nigra

a. Line of darker pigmentation extending from the pubis to the umbilicus in some women

b. Small, bright-red, vascular elevations of the skin often found on the chest, arms, legs, and neck

c. The "mask of pregnancy," an irregular pigmentation commonly found on the cheeks, forehead, and nose

d. Wavy, irregular, reddish streaks commonly found on the abdomen, breasts, or thighs; often referred to as "stretch marks"

29. A pregnant woman tells you that her friends tease her about her "stomach-first, waddling walk." She asks why she walks this way. How would you respond?

30. Briefly describe the functions of the following hormones in pregnancy:

    a. Human chorionic gonadotropin (hCG)

    b. Estrogen

    c. Progesterone

    d. Human placental lactogen (hPL)

    e. Relaxin

31. Describe the effects of pregnancy on the following components of the endocrine system:

    a. Thyroid

    b. Pancreas

    c. Pituitary

    d. Adrenals

32. Briefly discuss the proposed functions of prostaglandins during pregnancy.

33. What is the recommended weight gain for a woman of normal weight before pregnancy?

    _____

34. What is the average pattern of weight gain during each trimester of pregnancy?

    a. First trimester: _____

    b. Second trimester: _____

    c. Third trimester: _____

For each of the following signs of pregnancy, indicate with an **S**, **O**, *or* **D** *whether the sign is* <u>s</u>*ubjective (presumptive),* <u>o</u>*bjective (probable), or* <u>d</u>*iagnostic (positive)*

35. _____ Amenorrhea

36. _____ Goodell's sign

37. _____ Fetal heart sounds

38. _____ Urinary frequency

39. _____ Positive pregnancy test

40. _____ Nausea and vomiting

41. _____ Enlargement of the abdomen

42. _____ Quickening

43. _____ Palpable fetal movements

44. _____ Braxton Hicks contractions

45. How would you explain the differences among subjective (presumptive), objective (probable), and diagnostic (positive) signs of pregnancy to an expectant mother?

PREGNANCY TESTS

46. Briefly describe each of the following pregnancy tests:

    a. Hemagglutination-inhibition test

    b. Latex agglutination tests

    c. b-subunit radioimmunoassay (RIA)

    d. Enzyme-linked immunosorbent assay (ELISA)

    e. Immunoradiometric assay (IRMA)

    f. Fluoroimmunoassay (FIA)

47. Why is a positive pregnancy test *not* a positive sign of pregnancy?

48. Over-the-counter pregnancy tests determine the presence of hCG in the woman's

   a. blood.

   b. saliva.

   c. urine.

   d. vaginal secretions.

PSYCHOLOGIC RESPONSE OF THE EXPECTANT FAMILY TO PREGNANCY

49. Briefly summarize behaviors that are commonly seen in each trimester as a woman adjusts to pregnancy.

Trimester	Behaviors
First trimester	
Second trimester	
Third trimester	

50. Discuss the possible effects of pregnancy on a woman's body image.

REFLECTIONS

Think of some pregnant women you have known or cared for who were at different stages of pregnancy. How did their responses to pregnancy vary? What feelings did they describe? How did their partners react? Their parents? Other children in the family?

_____

_____

_____

_____

_____

_____

_____

51. According to Rubin (1984), a pregnant woman faces four main psychologic tasks as she works to maintain her intactness and that of her family while also preparing a place for her new child. Identify and briefly summarize these tasks.

a.

b.

c.

d.

52. As her pregnancy progresses, Alana Valdez begins to see less of the women in her Young Businesswomen's Club and spends more time with two neighbors who have young children. Which of Rubin's psychologic tasks of pregnancy is she attempting to complete?

    a. Ensuring safe passage through pregnancy, labor, and birth

    b. Seeking acceptance of this child by others

    c. Seeking commitment and acceptance of self as mother to the infant

    d. Learning to give of self on behalf of child

53. Your close friend has just received confirmation that she is 10 weeks pregnant. She tells you that she feels some ambivalence about being pregnant and having a child, even though the pregnancy was planned. How might you respond?

54. Like the pregnant woman, the expectant father's reactions to pregnancy tend to vary by trimester. For each trimester, describe the commonly occurring responses of the father.

    First trimester:

    Second trimester:

    Third trimester:

55. Briefly explain the concept of *couvade.*

56. Monica D'Angelo is 6 months pregnant and asks for advice about how to prepare her 3-year-old son Nicky for the birth of a sibling. What suggestions might you give her?

57. Imagine you are the head nurse in a prenatal clinic that provides care for women from a variety of ethnic backgrounds. You are responsible for orienting new nurses. Summarize three or four key points for the nurses to remember when caring for women from different cultures.

58. **Memory Check:** Define the following abbreviations.

   a. hCG

   b. hPL

CHAPTER 7

NURSING ASSESSMENT AND CARE OF THE EXPECTANT FAMILY

The antepartal period is a time of tremendous importance for the expectant family and their unborn child. During this time the family must adjust to the physical and psychologic changes occurring in the mother and also come to terms with the impact of a new baby on their own lives and roles in the family. In addition, fetal well-being is directly related to the mother's health, personal habits, and environment. This chapter corresponds to Chapters 15, 16, 17, and 18 in the eighth edition of *Olds' Maternal-Newborn Nursing & Women's Health Across the Lifespan*.

PRENATAL ASSESSMENT

1. What is the purpose of the initial client history?

MediaLink

http://www.prenhall.com/davidson

Additional resources for this content can be found on the Student DVD-ROM accompanying the eighth edition of *Olds' Maternal-Newborn Nursing & Women's Health Across the Lifespan* and on the Companion Website at http://www.prenhall.com/davidson. Click on the text chapter number(s) listed for this content to select the appropriate activities.

Prentice Hall Nursing MediaLink DVD-ROM
- Audio Glossary
- NCLEX Review
- Tools: Food Guide Pyramid
- Tools: RDAs for Females During Pregnancy and Lactation
- Tools: Maternal-Newborn Laboratory Values

Companion Website
- Additional NCLEX Review
- Case Study: Initial Prenatal Assessment
- Case Study: First Trimester Client
- Case Study: Adolescent Pregnancy
- Case Study: Maternal Weight Gain
- Care Plan Activity: Initial Assessment of Primigravida
- Care Plan Activity: Common Discomforts of Pregnancy
- Care Plan Activity: Adolescent Pregnancy
- Care Plan Activity: Maternal Nutrition
- Tools: Food Guide Pyramid
- Tools: RDAs for Females During Pregnancy and Lactation
- Tools: Maternal-Newborn Laboratory Values

Match the terms on the left, which are used when developing a woman's obstetric history, with the definitions on the right:

2. _____ Gravida

3. _____ Multipara

4. _____ Nulligravida

5. _____ Para

6. _____ Primigravida

a. A woman who has had two or more births at more than 20 weeks' gestation

b. A woman who has never been pregnant

c. A woman who is pregnant for the first time

d. Any pregnancy, regardless of its duration, including the present pregnancy

e. A woman who has not given birth at more than 20 weeks' gestation

f. Birth after 20 weeks' gestation, regardless of whether the infant is born alive or dead

7. Roya Siroospour is pregnant for the fourth time. She lost her first pregnancy at 12 weeks' gestation. She has two children at home. How would you record her obstetric history?

Gravida _____   Para _____   Ab _____   Living children _____

8. a. Yolanda Jackson is pregnant for the third time. She gave birth to a stillborn infant at 36 weeks' gestation and has a 3-year-old at home who was born at term. How would you record her obstetric history?

Gravida _____   Para _____   Ab _____   Living children _____

b. A more detailed approach can also be used. In this approach, the meaning of *gravida* remains unchanged, whereas *para* changes slightly to focus on the number of infants born. Use the acronym TPAL to remember *T*erm, *P*reterm, *A*bortions, *L*iving children. Using this method, how would you record Yolanda's obstetric history?

Gravida _____   Para _____   _____   _____   _____

9. The following questionnaire is similar to many that are used when a woman initially seeks antepartal care. With a friend or family member acting as the client and you as the prenatal nurse, obtain the necessary information. (Note: This questionnaire focuses primarily on factors related to pregnancy and is not a complete history of all body systems.)

Name: _____   Age: _____ Race: _____

Address: _____   Phone: _____

Educational level: _____   Occupation: _____

Marital status: _____   Religious preference (optional): _____

Have any members of your family had the following? If so, who?

_____ Diabetes_____

_____ Cardiovascular disease _____

_____ High blood pressure _____

_____ Breast cancer _____

_____ Other types of cancer _____

_____ Multiple pregnancies _____

_____ Preeclampsia-eclampsia _____

_____ Congenital anomalies _____

How old were you when your menstrual periods started? _____

How often do they occur? _____

How long do they last? _____

Do you have any discomfort with your periods? _____   If so, how severe is it? _____

What is the date of the first day of your last normal menstrual period? _____

Have you had any bleeding or spotting since your last normal menstrual period? _____

Have you had any of the following diseases?

_____ Chickenpox   _____ Asthma

_____ Mumps   _____ High blood pressure

_____ Three-day measles (rubella)   _____ Heart disease

_____ Two-week measles (rubeola)   _____ Respiratory disease

_____ Kidney disease   _____ Diabetes

_____ Frequent bladder infections   _____ Allergies

_____ Thyroid problems   _____ Sexually transmitted infection

_____ Anemia   _____ Other

(If the woman answers *yes* to any of the above, include pertinent information in this space.)

Have you been on birth control pills? _____   If yes, when did you stop taking them? _____

Were you using any other method of contraception? _____   If so, what method? _____

How many previous pregnancies have you had? _____

Have you had any miscarriages or abortions? _____   If yes, how many? _____

How many living children do you have? _____

Have you had any stillbirths? _____   If yes, how many? _____

Gravida _____   Para_____   Ab_____

Previous children:

	Date of birth	Sex	Birth weight	Preterm or full term
1.				
2.				
3.				
4.				
5.				

Did any previous children have problems immediately after birth? _____ If yes, what occurred?

Have you had any problems with previous pregnancies? _____ If yes, what occurred?

Have you had any problems with previous labors and/or births? _____ If yes, what occurred?

Have you had any problems with previous postpartal periods? _____ If yes, what occurred?

Are you presently taking any prescription or nonprescription drugs? _____ If yes, please list them:

Do you smoke? _____ Number of cigarettes per day: _____

How much of the following do you drink each day? Coffee _____ Tea _____

Colas _____ Alcoholic beverages _____

What is your present weight? _____ What is your usual prepregnant weight? _____

Nursing assessment of available psychosocial data *(to be completed by nurse using information obtained from the woman or other sources):*[1]

---

[1] This should be a brief summary of your impression of the woman, her ability to cope with her pregnancy, plans she has made, and available support systems.

Brief description of available support persons (include information about the father of the child such as age, occupation, involvement in the pregnancy):

Client's feelings about the pregnancy and her plans for dealing with it:

Does the client have any cultural or religious practices that might influence her care or that of her child?

For the prenatal laboratory test results in the following list, indicate with an **N** *if the result is normal or an* **A** *if the result is abnormal and requires further evaluation.*

10. _____ Hemoglobin 13.6 g/dL

11. _____ Hematocrit 35%

12. _____ Rubella titer 1:6

13. _____ WBC 6200/microliter

14. _____ Sickle cell screen negative

15. During the prenatal assessment, the woman is screened for risk factors. What are risk factors?

16. Give three examples of factors that increase a woman's risk during pregnancy.

a.

b.

c.

The procedure for a complete physical examination may be reviewed in textbooks on physical assessment. This workbook focuses on those aspects of the physical examination that are directly related to assessment of the pregnancy.

17. Jenny Nishida, gravida 1, para 0, ab 0, is scheduled for her first obstetric examination. Identify three areas of focus in this examination.

    a.

    b.

    c.

18. During her examination, the nurse practitioner (or physician) measures Jenny's fundal height. How is this measured?

19. a. What information does fundal height provide about the pregnancy?

    b. Where would you expect to find the fundus at 12 weeks' gestation? _____

    c. At 20 weeks' gestation? _____

20. Jenny asks you when the baby's heartbeat will be heard. When is the fetal heartbeat usually detected with a Doppler? _____

21. To complete a pelvic examination, Jenny is placed in the _____ position.

22. Identify the three basic parts of every initial pelvic examination.

    a.

    b.

    c.

23. If you noted on a prenatal record that a woman had a diagonal conjugate of 9 cm, what possible problems might you predict for her labor?

24. What is the purpose of Nägele's rule?

25. How is Nägele's rule calculated?

26. Jenny began her last normal menstrual period on March 22 of this year. Using Nägele's rule, calculate her expected date of birth (EDB).

27. What is the recommended frequency of prenatal visits for a normal prenatal client?

28. Identify the factors that you would consider part of your initial psychologic assessment of an antepartal family.

For each of the following warning signs, select a possible cause from the choices on the right. Use each answer only once.

29. _____ Dysuria   a. Preeclampsia

30. _____ Persistent vomiting   b. Placenta previa

31. _____ Abdominal pain   c. Urinary tract infection

32. _____ Epigastric pain   d. Hyperemesis gravidarum

33. _____ Vaginal bleeding   e. Abruptio placentae

34. What would you instruct a woman to do if she experiences any of the danger signs in pregnancy?

COMMON DISCOMFORTS OF PREGNANCY

35. From the list that follows, circle the discomforts that commonly occur during the first trimester of pregnancy:

    varicose veins, urinary frequency, nausea and vomiting,

    backache, dyspnea, flatulence, fatigue, leg cramps,

    breast tenderness, faintness, increased vaginal discharge

36. For each of the following discomforts, identify at least one self-care measure a pregnant woman might use to obtain relief:

    a. Breast tenderness

    b. Leg cramps

    c. Nausea

    d. Constipation

    e. Backache

    f. Urinary frequency

37. Your friend is in her early months of pregnancy and complains about morning sickness. Which of the following recommendations might you make to her?

    a. Nothing will alleviate it, and you must do your best to accept it.

    b. Eat a dry carbohydrate, such as crackers, before arising.

    c. Take large quantities of fluids with meals.

    d. Eat three meals per day and avoid eating between meals.

38. **Critical Thinking in Practice:** The following action sequence is designed to help you think through basic clinical problems. Read the sequence, then fill in the appropriate boxes in the flowchart on page 62.

    Julie Dombrowski, gravida 1, para 0, is 12 weeks pregnant when she comes for her second prenatal visit. She tells you that her main problem is noticeable fatigue. She states, "Sometimes I'm so tired by the end of the day that I can hardly make it home to cook supper. I can't tell you how many meals Larry has cooked lately because I don't have the energy to do it. Is something wrong with me?"

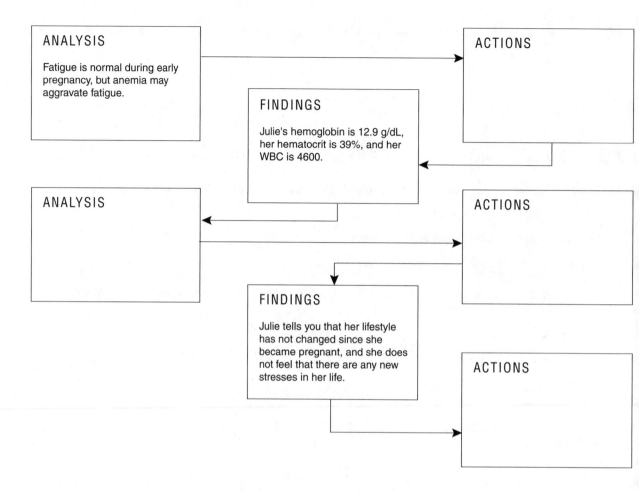

ANALYSIS

Fatigue is normal during early pregnancy, but anemia may aggravate fatigue.

ACTIONS

FINDINGS

Julie's hemoglobin is 12.9 g/dL, her hematocrit is 39%, and her WBC is 4600.

ANALYSIS

ACTIONS

FINDINGS

Julie tells you that her lifestyle has not changed since she became pregnant, and she does not feel that there are any new stresses in her life.

ACTIONS

TEACHING FOR SELF-CARE DURING PREGNANCY

39. Theresa Rashid works as an accountant for a large firm and dresses professionally. She asks you if she can continue to wear high heels to work. How would you respond?

40. Theresa asks about the types of physical activity she can engage in during pregnancy. What guidelines would you suggest she follow when engaging in sports and physical activities?

41. Several approaches to tracking fetal activity exist and are often referred to as a fetal movement record or fetal activity diary. Describe the procedure for tracking fetal activity that is used in your clinical facility.

42. What advice would you give a pregnant woman who states that she is a "bath person" and prefers tub baths to showers?

43. Linh Trang, 7 months pregnant, asks about traveling 300 miles by car to visit her parents. Her pregnancy, to date, is normal. What advice would you give her?

44. The pregnant woman should have a dental examination (a) _____ in her pregnancy. Dental x-rays should be (b) _____.

45. What advice would you give a woman 11 weeks pregnant who asks about having an occasional glass of wine during her pregnancy?

46. Kathy Markowitz is 7 months pregnant with her first child. She tells you that she and her partner, Yakov, still find sexual intercourse very satisfying, although recently they have found it more comfortable to make love if Kathy assumes the superior position. Kathy says that she and Yakov recently talked about making love during the last weeks of pregnancy. They wondered if it was "okay" or if it posed a threat for Kathy or the baby. After assessing Kathy's concerns, formulate an appropriate nursing diagnosis.

47. A substance that adversely affects the normal growth and development of the fetus is called a

_____.

AGE-RELATED CONSIDERATIONS

48. Identify three advantages of delaying childbirth until a woman is in her 30s.

    a.

    b.

    c.

49. A child born to a woman over age 35 has an increased risk of

    a. cleft palate.

    b. cystic fibrosis.

    c. Down syndrome.

    d. meningomyelocele.

50. In addition to concerns about the baby's well-being and the health of the mother, identify three concerns that many couples face when they delay childbearing until the mother is in her 30s.

    a.

    b.

    c.

ADOLESCENT PREGNANCY

51. Identify at least six reasons why an adolescent might become pregnant.

    a.

    b.

    c.

d.

e.

f.

52. Imagine you are responsible for developing a prenatal clinic for adolescent girls. What factors about the adolescent and her development would you consider in planning your approach? Identify some specific techniques or services you would like to have available for the adolescent.

53. Pregnant adolescents are at high risk for certain complications. From the list that follows, circle those medical or pregnancy-related complications that occur most commonly in pregnant adolescents: iron deficiency anemia, urinary tract infection, diabetes mellitus, preeclampsia, preterm birth, macrosomia, cephalopelvic disproportion (CPD), multiple gestation.

MATERNAL NUTRITION

54. Nina Suh, a 22-year-old primipara who is 2 months pregnant, is discussing nutrition with you. She is of normal weight and is very concerned about avoiding excessive weight gain. What pattern of weight gain would you recommend for her?

55. To achieve this weight gain, she should increase her daily intake by _____ kcal.

56. Which of the following menus would provide the highest amounts of protein, iron, and vitamin C?

    a. 4 oz beef, 1/2 c lima beans, a glass of skim milk, and 3/4 c strawberries

    b. 3 oz chicken, 1/2 c corn, a lettuce salad, and a small banana

    c. 1 c macaroni, 3/4 c peas, a glass of whole milk, and a medium pear

    d. A scrambled egg, hashbrown potatoes, half a glass of buttermilk, and a large nectarine

REFLECTIONS

Think about any pregnant adolescents you have cared for as a nursing student or have known. Compare their reactions to being pregnant to those of more mature pregnant women. How are they similar? Different?

_____

_____

_____

_____

_____

_____

_____

_____

For each of the vitamins or minerals in the following list, select the answer that best describes their function from the column on the right.

57. _____ Vitamin A

58. _____ Vitamin E

59. _____ Vitamin K

60. _____ Vitamin C

61. _____ Folic acid

62. _____ Pyridoxine (B_6)

63. _____ Calcium

64. _____ Zinc

65. _____ Magnesium

a. Prevents night blindness

b. Necessary for normal blood clotting

c. Essential to formation of connective tissue

d. Synthesis of DNA and RNA

e. Amino acid metabolism

f. Cellular metabolism

g. Deficiency associated with neural tube defects

h. Mineralization of fetal bones and teeth

i. Antioxidation

66. Gloria Ristow is a true vegetarian and will not eat any food from animal sources, including milk and eggs. What foods might she use to meet her protein and calcium requirements during pregnancy?

67. The following is a 24-hour food diary for a 26-year-old pregnant woman of normal weight. Analyze its adequacy with regard to the basic food groups.

    Breakfast:

    3/4 oz dry cereal

    1/2 cup lowfat milk

    4 oz orange juice

    Lunch:

    sandwich made with 2 slices whole wheat bread, 2 oz chicken breast, lettuce, mayonnaise

    8 oz milk

    1 small chocolate bar

    Dinner:

    6 oz flounder

    tossed salad with dressing

    1/2 cup rice

    1 piece of cake

    Snack:

    1 1/2 cup vanilla ice cream

    Analysis:

    Dairy products:

    Meat group:

    Grains:

    Fruits and vegetables:

68. **Memory Check:** Define the following abbreviations.

   a. EDB

   b. EDC

   c. EDD

   d. FAD

   e. FMR

   f. G

   g. P

   h. RDA

CHAPTER 8

PREGNANCY AT RISK: PREGESTATIONAL PROBLEMS

An at-risk pregnancy is one in which certain factors or groups of factors increase the possibility of illness, harm, or even death to the mother and/or the fetus (or newborn). This chapter focuses on preexisting conditions, such as substance abuse or maternal heart disease, that cause a pregnancy to be considered at risk. This chapter corresponds to Chapter 19 in the eighth edition of *Olds' Maternal-Newborn Nursing & Women's Health Across the Lifespan*.

SUBSTANCE ABUSE AND PREGNANCY

1. Statistically, approximately _____ out of _____ women in the United States currently is abusing a substance.

2. From the list that follows, circle those signs or symptoms that are commonly seen in the newborns of women who have abused crack or cocaine:

   Exaggerated startle response, genitourinary malformations, hydrocephalus, increased risk of sudden infant death syndrome (SIDS), intrauterine growth restriction (IUGR), marked passivity, shorter body length

3. Elizabeth Ivanovna, 4 months pregnant with her first child, is seen for her first prenatal visit. During her initial history she admits that she uses cocaine regularly. As her nurse, identify at least three areas of assessment you should focus on in caring for her.

   a.

   b.

   c.

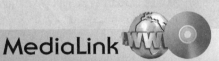

MediaLink

http://www.prenhall.com/davidson

Additional resources for this content can be found on the Student DVD-ROM accompanying the eighth edition of *Olds' Maternal-Newborn Nursing & Women's Health Across the Lifespan,* and on the Companion Website at http://www.prenhall.com/davidson. Click on the text chapter number(s) listed for this content to select the appropriate activities.

Prentice Hall Nursing MediaLink DVD-ROM
- Audio Glossary
- NCLEX Review

Companion Website
- Additional NCLEX Review
- Case Study: Client with Gestational Diabetes
- Care Plan Activity: Antepartal Client at Risk

4. What methods of pain relief are best for Elizabeth during her labor? _____

_____

5. True or False _____: Pain medication should never be administered to a laboring woman who is a

substance abuser. Why? _____

_____

DIABETES MELLITUS AND PREGNANCY

6. The four cardinal signs and symptoms of diabetes are:

a. _____   c. _____

b. _____   d. _____

7. Myrna Lerudis is pregnant for the second time. Her first child weighed 9 lb, 11 oz. Her doctors perform a glucose tolerance test and discover elevated blood glucose levels. Because Myrna shows no signs of diabetes when she is not pregnant, she is best classified as having

a. type 1 diabetes mellitus.

b. type 2 diabetes mellitus.

c. gestational diabetes mellitus.

d. secondary diabetes mellitus.

8. Following birth, the infant of a woman with preexisting diabetes mellitus (White's classes A, B, or C) is at greatest risk for the development of

a. anemia.

b. hypercalcemia.

c. hyperglycemia.

d. hypoglycemia.

9. Identify three ways in which pregnancy can affect diabetes.

a.

b.

c.

10. Identify four maternal and/or fetal complications that may occur during pregnancy as a result of diabetes mellitus.

a. _____   c. _____

b. _____   d. _____

11. **Critical Thinking Challenge:** The following situation has been included to challenge your critical thinking. Read the situation and then answer "yes" or "no" to the question that follows.

    Belle Cavillo, a 29-year-old gravida 2, para 1, was diagnosed as having diabetes mellitus a year ago. Her diabetes was controlled with low doses of insulin. When her pregnancy was diagnosed at 7 weeks' gestation, her glycosylated hemoglobin was 6.4% and her fasting blood glucose (FBG) was 98 mg/dL. Belle missed her last two prenatal visits but states that she carefully followed her diet and insulin dosage schedule. Today's FBG is 96 mg/dL and her glycosylated hemoglobin is 7%.

    Did Belle maintain effective control?

    Yes _____   No _____

    Explain your answer:

12. You ask Belle if she can think of anything that would make it easier for her to keep her appointments. She states, "There is a satellite clinic really close to my house, but they won't see me because they say I'm high risk." You know that Belle's physician works at that clinic 1 day a week. You explain the situation to Belle's doctor and ask her if she would be willing to see Belle there. The physician agrees, and Belle is delighted with the change. Evaluate the effectiveness of your intervention.

13. Isadora Filatov has newly diagnosed gestational diabetes and is started on insulin in four doses, one before each meal and one at bedtime. She asks why four shots are necessary. How would you respond?

14. What advice would you give Isadora about continuing her regular exercise program?

15. Is breastfeeding safe for women with diabetes?

    a. yes

    b. no

16. A friend of yours is diagnosed as having gestational diabetes. She tells you that her grandmother takes a pill for diabetes. Your friend asks why she can't simply take something by mouth, too. What would you tell her?

17. Your friend also asks why infants of diabetic mothers are often large at birth. How would you explain this phenomenon?

18. List three tests that might be performed to assess fetal status in a pregnant woman with diabetes.

    a.

    b.

    c.

19. In broad terms, the two primary causes of anemia in pregnancy are

    a.

    b.

20. _____ anemia is the most common complication of pregnancy.

21. Briefly describe the pathophysiology of sickle cell anemia and its potential impact on the pregnant woman and on her fetus/newborn.

HIV INFECTION AND PREGNANCY

22. HIV infection from mother to fetus can occur during pregnancy. HIV may also be transmitted to the newborn in breast milk. However, maternal transmission of infection most commonly occurs _____.

23. Identify four signs of developing complications in a pregnant HIV-positive woman.

a. _____   c. _____

b. _____   d. _____

24. In caring for any pregnant woman, when should gloves be worn?

REFLECTIONS

HIV/AIDS is a devastating diagnosis for childbearing women and their loved ones. How do you feel about caring for families with HIV/AIDS? Do you have any preconceived views? Take a few moments to reflect on your own beliefs and attitudes. Do they influence the care you give?

_____

_____

_____

_____

_____

_____

_____

HEART DISEASE AND PREGNANCY

25. The New York Heart Association classification of functional capacity is used to assess the severity of cardiac disease. For each of the classes, state the expected physical activity level.

    a. Class I

    b. Class II

    c. Class III

    d. Class IV

26. Sandy Meltzner is a 24-year-old woman who is classified as a class III cardiac client. List five signs and symptoms that would lead you to suspect cardiac decompensation in Sandy.

    a.

    b.

    c.

    d.

    e.

27. Juanita Alvarez has a history of cardiac problems following an episode of rheumatic fever. She experiences dyspnea and palpitations when she bicycles around her neighborhood. Which classification of functional capacity best applies?

    a. Class I

    b. Class II

    c. Class III

    d. Class IV

28. Which of the following statements about the nutritional needs of pregnant women with a cardiac condition is most accurate?

    a. They require major increases in iron and calories but decreased sodium.

    b. They require increased protein and iron but minimized sodium intake.

    c. They require optimal amounts of all essential vitamins but restricted caloric and iron intake.

    d. They require increased iron, protein, sodium, carbohydrates, and fats.

29. Amy Chang, 10 weeks pregnant, is seen for her first prenatal visit. She had rheumatic fever as a child and is currently classified as a class II cardiac client. In addition to iron and vitamin supplements, Amy has been started on penicillin. She asks you why this was done. What would you tell her?

30. In the absence of complications, what is the method of choice by which Amy would give birth?

31. **Memory Check:** Define the following abbreviations.

   a. AIDS

   b. DM

   c. FAS

   d. GDM

   e. HIV

   f. IDDM

CHAPTER 9

PREGNANCY AT RISK: GESTATIONAL ONSET

Most pregnancies proceed without difficulty. Occasionally, however, complications develop that increase the risk for the pregnant woman and/or the fetus (or newborn). This chapter focuses on problems, such as bleeding or preeclampsia, that have their onset during pregnancy. It corresponds to Chapter 20 in the eighth edition of *Olds' Maternal-Newborn Nursing & Women's Health Across the Lifespan.*

BLEEDING DISORDERS

1. Define *spontaneous abortion.*

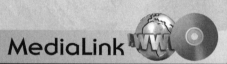

MediaLink

http://www.prenhall.com/davidson

Additional resources for this content can be found on the Student DVD-ROM accompanying the eighth edition of *Olds' Maternal-Newborn Nursing & Women's Health Across the Lifespan,* and on the Companion Website at http://www.prenhall.com/davidson. Click on the text chapter number(s) listed for this content to select the appropriate activities.

Prentice Hall Nursing MediaLink DVD-ROM
- Audio Glossary
- NCLEX Review

Companion Website
- Additional NCLEX Review
- Case Study: Client with Preeclampsia
- Care Plan Activity: Client at Risk for Preterm Labor

2. Spontaneous abortion may also be called _____.

Match the following terms with the correct definitions.

3. _____ Threatened abortion

4. _____ Imminent abortion

5. _____ Complete abortion

6. _____ Incomplete abortion

7. _____ Missed abortion

8. _____ Habitual abortion

a. Loss of three or more successive pregnancies

b. Abortion characterized by vaginal bleeding and cramping but a closed cervical os

c. Abortion in which the fetus dies in utero but is not expelled

d. Abortion in which all the products of conception are expelled

e. Abortion characterized by bleeding, cramping, and dilatation of the cervical os

f. Abortion in which a portion of the products of conception is retained

9. Alys Nandreya, a 22-year-old gravida 1, para 0, who is 11 weeks pregnant, was admitted to the hospital with moderate vaginal bleeding and some abdominal cramping. Vaginal examination reveals that the cervix is dilated 2 cm. She is diagnosed as having an imminent abortion. Identify four nursing interventions that are indicated in caring for Alys.

    a.

    b.

    c.

    d.

10. Alys is placed on bed rest with intravenous fluids and that evening passes some of the products of conception. The following morning she has a dilation and curettage (D&C). Why is this done?

11. Alys's husband asks you why abortions occur. Identify four causes of spontaneous abortion.

    a.

    b.

    c.

    d.

12. **Nursing Care Plan in Action:** For the following case scenario, focus on the pertinent data, formulate one appropriate nursing diagnosis, and complete all components of the nursing care plan.

    Case Scenario: Althea Stravinsky is a 26-year-old who is pregnant after trying for 2 years. She is 14 weeks' gestation. Althea and Oscar took pregestational and early prenatal classes. At each of the prenatal visits, they listen to the fetal heartbeat and both carry ultrasound pictures of "their baby." Althea is now seen in the clinic for vaginal spotting and mild abdominal cramping. Althea is crying and clinging to her husband's hand. She asks you why this is happening. Did she do something wrong? Her husband struggles to tell Althea that things will be okay.

NURSING CARE PLAN

Collaborative problems:

Nursing diagnosis:

Defining characteristics:

Goals: Client/husband will:

Interventions	Rationale	Expected Outcome
Assessments:		
Nursing Interventions:		
Collaborative:		

13. The most common cause of second trimester abortion is incompetent cervix. Identify two factors that may contribute to incompetent cervix.

    a.

    b.

14. A surgical procedure used to treat incompetent cervix so that a woman may successfully carry a pregnancy to term is _____.

15. Define *ectopic pregnancy.*

16. The most common implantation site in an ectopic pregnancy is the_____.

17. Ectopic pregnancy is often difficult to diagnose because its symptoms are similar to those of abdominal conditions. Identify at least five signs or symptoms of ectopic pregnancy and briefly explain why each occurs.

Sign or Symptom	Physiologic Rationale for Occurrence
a.	
b.	
c.	
d.	
e.	

18. Which of the following signs would *not* be indicative of a ruptured tubal pregnancy?

    a. Increased pulse and decreased blood pressure

    b. Marked lower abdominal pain

    c. Vaginal bleeding

    d. Urinary frequency

19. Which of the following findings would best support a diagnosis of gestational trophoblastic disease?

    a. Brownish vaginal discharge, hyperemesis gravidarum, absence of fetal heart tones

    b. Elevated human chorionic gonadotropin (hCG) levels, enlarged abdomen, quickening

    c. Vaginal bleeding, absence of fetal heart tones, decreased hCG levels

    d. Visible fetal skeleton with sonography, absence of quickening, enlarged abdomen

20. Lisa Chan is diagnosed as having gestational trophoblastic disease. Following successful removal of the molar pregnancy, Lisa is advised to avoid pregnancy for a year and to return for periodic measurement of hCG levels. What is the rationale for this advice?

HYPEREMESIS GRAVIDARUM

21. Define *hyperemesis gravidarum.*

22. Identify the goals of therapy if hospitalization becomes necessary because of hyperemesis gravidarum during pregnancy.

    a.

    b.

    c.

    d.

PREMATURE RUPTURE OF THE MEMBRANES (PROM)

23. Define *preterm PROM.*

24. The most common neonatal complication of preterm PROM is _____

    _____.

25. The greatest risk of PROM for the pregnant woman is _____.

26. Fill in the following blanks: When PROM is suspected, the fluid can be tested using _____.

    It turns _____in the presence of amniotic fluid, which is more _____

    (alkaline or acidic?) than normal vaginal secretions.

27. Michelle Niyompong has been hospitalized for preterm PROM. Her fluid has stopped leaking and she is being discharged. Identify at least four issues you should address with Michelle in completing her discharge teaching.

    a.

    b.

    c.

    d.

PRETERM LABOR

Sarah Benitah is 36 years old and is a gravida 4. She has two children at home; one was born at 35 weeks' gestation. Sarah has also had one spontaneous abortion. She smokes 15 cigarettes a day and has an occasional glass of wine. Sarah has a history of pyelonephritis. She has been working for the past 2 years in a factory. She provides the sole financial support for the family. Her job requires that she stand in one place along a conveyor belt and inspect parts as they pass by. Sarah had a brief episode of vaginal bleeding at 14 weeks' gestation, which lasted 2 days. Since then, the pregnancy has gone well; however, she has noted more contractions lately.

28. In the preceding narrative, circle all of Sarah's risk factors for preterm labor.

29. Sarah asks you what she should look for this time. Identify important information to include in your answer.

30. Sarah receives your information in a serious, thoughtful manner. At the end of your conversation, she says, "But how do I know if it's a real contraction?" How would you respond?

There are many signs and symptoms associated with preterm labor. When any of the signs and symptoms of preterm labor are present, it is important for the woman to call her healthcare provider and be evaluated in a healthcare birth setting. Place a "Y" beside all factors in the following list that would need further evaluation and an "N" beside those that are essentially normal.

31. _____ pinkish-colored vaginal discharge

32. _____ diarrhea

33. _____ thirst

34. _____ cramps in legs

35. _____ headache (mild) relieved by resting and cool cloth to forehead

36. _____ backache

37. _____ unusual tiredness

38. _____ increased appetite

39. Mrs. Benitah is admitted in preterm labor at 30 weeks' gestation and is started on intravenous magnesium sulfate. How does this medication work to control preterm labor?

40. The normal loading dose of magnesium sulfate in treating preterm labor is (a) _____ g in 100 mL solution per infusion pump over 15 to 20 minutes. The maintenance dose is (b) _____ g/hr per infusion pump.

41. The antagonist of magnesium sulfate is _____.

42. When magnesium sulfate is administered, careful nursing assessments are indicated. Identify at least five nursing assessments, the findings that would require further nursing action, and the rationale for each:

Assessment and Findings Requiring Further Action	Rationale

43. **Critical Thinking Challenge:** The following situation has been included to challenge your critical thinking. Read the situation and then answer the question "yes" or "no."

Helen Polawski is admitted to the birthing unit, and you will be responsible for her care. She is a gravida 4, para 3, ab 0, with three living children, one term birth, and two preterm births. She is at 34 weeks' gestation and is having contractions every 3 minutes of 40 seconds duration. She states that her membranes have been ruptured since yesterday at noon (23 hours ago). In your initial assessments, you find FHR 140, T 99.2, P 92, R 18, cervical dilatation 5 cm, and Nitrazine positive.

Is Helen a candidate for treatment to stop labor?

Yes _____   No _____

Explain your answer:

44. Ramona Aguilar is admitted in preterm labor at 32 weeks' gestation. In the first few minutes of care, many nursing actions are needed. Rank the nursing actions in order of priority. Place NA (not applicable) by those actions that could be deleted at this time.

   a. _____ Apply electronic monitor to determine contraction frequency and duration and FHR.

   b. _____ Assess maternal BP, TPR.

   c. _____ Complete all sections of the admission form.

   d. _____ Do a sterile vaginal examination to determine dilatation, effacement, fetal station, presentation, and position.

   e. _____ Use Nitrazine to test for ruptured membranes.

   f. _____ Weigh Ramona.

   g. _____ Listen to breath sounds.

PREECLAMPSIA AND ECLAMPSIA

45. **Critical Thinking in Practice:** The following action sequence is designed to help you think through clinical problems.

   You work as a professional nurse in a private obstetrician's office. Rita Sherbo, gravida 1, para 0, 37 weeks pregnant, is in for her weekly prenatal appointment. When you weigh her you note that she has gained 2¾ lb since last week. Her pregnancy to date has been completely normal. You know that the average weight gain in the last trimester is about 1 lb per week. A large weight gain often indicates that fluid is being retained. You know that this is an early sign of preeclampsia.

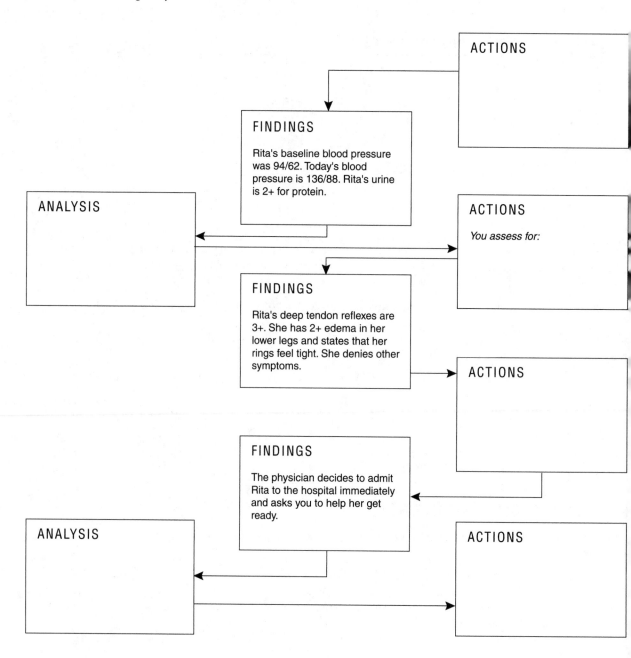

46. On the following chart, compare the signs and symptoms of mild preeclampsia and severe preeclampsia.

Sign	Mild Preeclampsia	Severe Preeclampsia
Blood pressure		
Weight gain		

(continued)

Sign	Mild Preeclampsia	Severe Preeclampsia
Edema		
Proteinuria		
Hyperreflexia		
Headache		
Epigastric pain		
Visual disturbances		

47. What additional symptom characterizes a woman as having eclampsia rather than severe preeclampsia?

   _____.

48. Women with a diagnosis of severe preeclampsia have an increased risk of

   a. complete abortion.

   b. placenta previa.

   c. abruptio placentae.

   d. none of the above.

49. Rita Sherbo is hospitalized with severe preeclampsia. Identify five interventions commonly used in caring for a woman with preeclampsia and the rationale for each.

Intervention	Rationale
a.	
b.	

Intervention	Rationale
c.	
d.	
e.	

50. You are administering intravenous magnesium sulfate to a woman with severe preeclampsia. You assess her and find her respirations are 12, her deep tendon reflexes (DTRs) are absent, and her urine output for the past 4 hours is 90 mL. What would you do?

    a. Administer calcium gluconate immediately.

    b. Administer only half the dose of magnesium sulfate.

    c. Continue the magnesium sulfate as ordered.

    d. Stop the magnesium sulfate and notify the doctor.

51. Your client, diagnosed with severe preeclampsia, is started on magnesium sulfate intravenously. In treating preeclampsia, the normal loading dose of magnesium sulfate is (a) _____ g given via infusion pump over (b) _____ minutes. The maintenance dose is (c) _____ g/hour via infusion pump.

52. Three signs of magnesium toxicity are (a) _____, (b) _____, and (c) _____.

53. HELLP syndrome is a major complication of preeclampsia-eclampsia. What do the letters HELLP stand for?
    H _____ E _____ L _____ L _____ P _____

54. Deborah Hermann is admitted to the birthing center in active labor with her first pregnancy. Her blood pressure is now 140/86 (blood pressure at first prenatal visit was 110/66); she has 2+ pitting edema in her feet, ankles, and lower legs; and she says that she has gained 4 lb over the last 2 days. You check her patellar deep tendon reflexes (DTRs). What does 3+ DTR mean?

55. As you check her DTRs, you also assess for clonus. How will you do this? What does two beats of clonus mean?

RH INCOMPATIBILITY

56. **Critical Thinking Challenge:** The following situation has been developed to challenge your critical thinking. Read the situation and then answer the question "yes" or "no."

    Your client, Carolyn Lorenzo, a gravida 2, para 2, is Rh−; her partner is Rh+. Her first child was Rh− . She has just given birth to an Rh+ infant. Her indirect Coombs' test is positive. Her infant's direct Coombs' test is also positive.

    Is Carolyn a candidate for Rh immune globulin (RhoGAM)?

    Yes _____   No _____

    Explain your answer:

57. What does Rh immune globulin do?

58. Briefly summarize the major risks for a woman and her fetus if the woman suffers trauma from an automobile accident during pregnancy.

INFECTIONS AND PREGNANCY

59. Thrush in the newborn is directly related to contact in the birth canal with which of the following organisms?

    a. *Candida albicans*

    b. *Neisseria gonorrhoeae*

    c. *Treponema pallidum*

    d. *Staphylococcus aureus*

60. In order to protect her unborn child from toxoplasmosis, a pregnant woman should

    a. avoid contact with people known to have German measles.

    b. avoid eating inadequately cooked meat.

    c. avoid sexual relations with known carriers of the causative organism.

    d. be vaccinated against it early in her pregnancy.

61. Exposure to rubella during the _____ trimester is the time of greatest risk for teratogenic effects in the fetus.

Match the maternal infections in the following list with the possible implications for the fetus or the pregnancy.

62. _____ Bacterial vaginosis

63. _____ Chlamydial infection

64. _____ Gonorrhea

65. _____ Syphilis

a. If untreated, newborn may develop pneumonia or conjunctivitis.

b. Risk of congenital infection or a stillborn infant.

c. If infection is present at time of birth, newborn may develop ophthalmia neonatorum.

d. Increased risk of PROM and preterm birth.

66. Saulia Grebliunas, pregnant with her first child, has a history of genital herpes simplex virus. She tells you that she has heard that her baby can become infected by the virus and had expected to have a cesarean. However, her physician has told her that it is too soon to know the method of birth. She asks you why it is too soon. How would you explain it to her?

67. Currently, the Centers for Disease Control and Prevention (CDC) recommends screening for group B streptococcal (GBS) infection at 35 to 37 weeks' gestation for which of the following?

a. All pregnant women

b. Women with a history of GBS

c. Women whose partners have been diagnosed with GBS

d. Women with existing GBS

68. **Memory Check:** Define the following abbreviations.

a. CID

d. DTR

b. CMV

e. STD

c. DIC

f. STI

CHAPTER 10

ASSESSMENT OF FETAL WELL-BEING

Nurses have an important role in fetal assessment. The nurse frequently provides the one-on-one teaching regarding the purpose, procedure, and possible alternatives of each fetal test. This chapter addresses the diagnostic testing that may be done during the prenatal period.

This chapter corresponds to Chapter 21 in the eighth edition of *Olds' Maternal-Newborn Nursing & Women's Health Across the Lifespan.*

ULTRASOUND

1. Ultrasound can be used for all of the following in the first trimester except

   a. establishing gestational age.

   b. assistance with CVS or nuchal translucency testing (ntt).

   c. guidance for amniocentesis.

   d. determining the presence of twins.

2. List two advantages for the mother and fetus of using ultrasound for assessment.

   a.

   b.

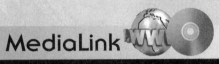

3. Identify at least six uses of ultrasound during early and late pregnancy.

Early Pregnancy (to 24 weeks)	Late Pregnancy (over 30 weeks)
a.	
b.	
c.	
d.	
e.	
f.	

4. Mrs. Michael Jacks is having an ultrasound examination. She asks, "Is it safe for my baby?" What will you say?

5. Sherry Adams, gravida 3, para 1, is in her 23rd week of pregnancy. Her last normal menstrual period began 5 1/2 months ago, but she had some bleeding 4 1/2 months ago. Your physical assessment provides the following data: The fundus is palpable at two fingerbreadths below the umbilicus; the fetal heart rate (FHR) is 140. Sherry states that she has not felt quickening. Based on this information, why do you think Sherry will have an ultrasound done?

6. Sherry asks you what is involved in having an ultrasound. How will you respond?

7. Latonya James is a 36-year-old G1P0 who wishes to have a nuchal translucency test. She is concerned about the risk of fetal loss with an amniocentesis. All of the following are true except

   a. it is a diagnostic test.

   b. it is a screening test.

   c. it screens for Trisomies, 13, 18, and 21.

   d. it cannot screen for neural tube defects.

MATERNAL ASSESSMENT OF FETAL ACTIVITY

8. Carla Cortez is pregnant for the first time. She asks you how to monitor her baby's movements.

   a. Write out your teaching plan. On a separate sheet of paper, devise a score sheet that she could use.

   b. She asks if there is anything she can do that might affect the number of movements. How will you answer?

NONSTRESS TESTING

9. What is the function of a nonstress test (NST)?

10. Explain the procedure for performing an NST.

11. Fetal heart rate patterns in NSTs have three classifications. Describe what a fetal monitoring strip would show in each case. What further testing may be indicated?

    a. Reactive

    b. Nonreactive

    c. Unsatisfactory

12. What is the best test result? Why?

13. Label each section of Figure 10–1, *A* and *B* as reactive, nonreactive, or unsatisfactory.

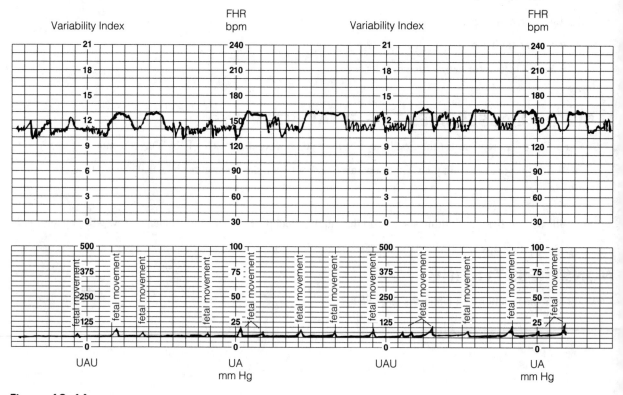

Figure 10–1A _____

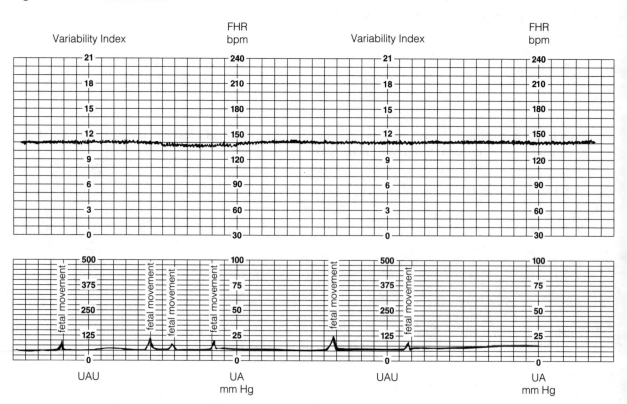

Figure 10–1B _____

14. The NST can be modified by adding a vibroacoustic stimulation (VAS) test. Describe how the VAS changes the basic NST.

BIOPHYSICAL PROFILE

15. A biophysical profile is completed to assess the fetus.

    a. Discuss the five specific areas assessed in this test.

    b. How is it scored? What represents a "desirable" or "good" score?

    c. Describe the conditions in which it is most likely for a fetal biophysical profile to be done.

    d. What does a decreased amniotic fluid volume mean?

    e. Bob Caplan calls the birth center and says, "My wife is to have a fetal biophysical profile tomorrow. What is it?" Write out how you will describe the assessment test to him.

CONTRACTION STRESS TESTING

16. List two indications for doing a contraction stress test (CST). Describe the physiologic rationale behind each indication.

    a.

    b.

17. List three *contraindications* for the CST. Describe the physiologic rationale behind each.

18. Describe the procedure for the breast self-stimulation test (BSST).

19. Explain the major differences between BSST and CST with intravenous oxytocin (sometimes called oxytocin challenge test).

Match the CST results with their corresponding definitions.

20. _____ Positive

21. _____ Negative

a. Late decelerations occur with 50% or more of the uterine contractions

b. No late decelerations occur with a minimum of three uterine contractions (lasting 40 to 60 seconds) in a 10-minute window.

22. a. Label the CST tracing in Figure 10–2 as positive or negative.

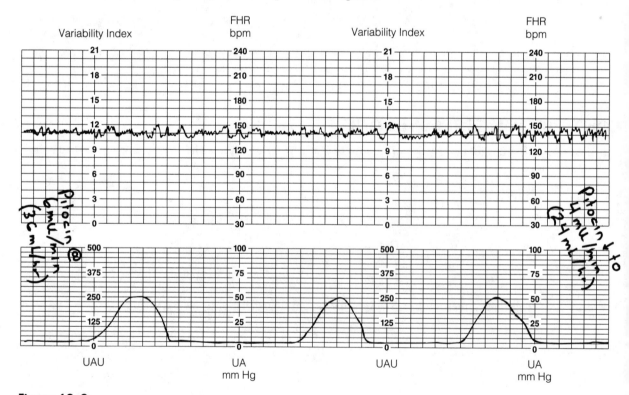

Figure 10–2 _____

b. What factors led you to this conclusion?

23. On the tracing in Figure 10–3, draw your own test results. Use different colored ink so the tracings will stand out.

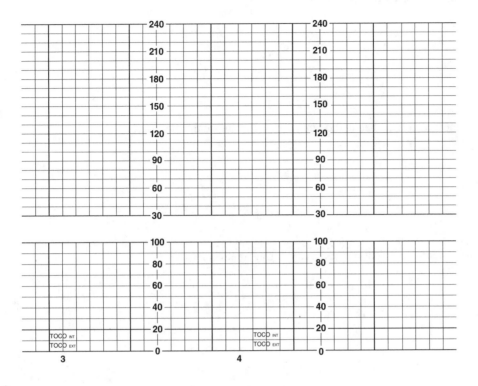

Figure 10–3

MATERNAL SERUM ALPHA-FETOPROTEIN (MSAFP) TESTING

24. Nancy Danforth is a 26-year-old, gravida 2, para 1. She asks you what the "quadruple check" screens for? You tell her it screens for all of the following except

  a. Down syndrome.

  b. trisomy 18.

  c. neural tube defects.

  d. cleft palate.

CHORIONIC VILLI SAMPLING

25. Amanda Rothstein is a 45-year-old gravida 1, para 0, who conceived after in vitro fertilization (IVF). She is 8 weeks pregnant and asks you the difference between chorionic villi sampling (CVS) and an amniocentesis. What is your response?

AMNIOCENTESIS

26. What is the purpose of amniocentesis?

27. Before amniocentesis, what method may be used to locate the placenta?

28. List three nursing interventions necessary during amniocentesis.

    a.

    b.

    c.

REFLECTIONS

Talk with a pregnant woman who is having prenatal testing done. What are her needs, concerns, and fears? Does she understand the reason for the test and what the test results mean? Does she know what to expect? What advice does she have for nurses who work in the antepartal testing situation?

_____

_____

_____

_____

_____

_____

29. List three complications associated with amniocentesis and the cause of each complication.

    a. _____   c. _____

    b. _____

FETAL LUNG MATURITY

30. Complete the chart on various tests that may be performed on amniotic fluid in the later portion of pregnancy.

Test	Purpose of Test	Normal Results	What Results Mean
Lecithin/sphingomyelin ratio (L/S)			
Phosphatidylglycerol			

31. **Critical Thinking in Practice:** The following action sequence is designed to help you think through clinical problems.

Yolanda King, a 37-year-old primipara, had an amniocentesis today. Yolanda calls the antepartal testing room 5 hours after her amniocentesis and says she is having contractions. Yolanda is at 38 weeks' gestation.

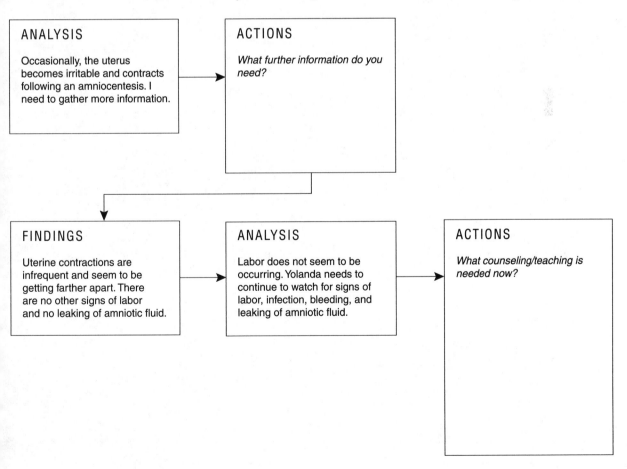

ANALYSIS

Occasionally, the uterus becomes irritable and contracts following an amniocentesis. I need to gather more information.

ACTIONS

What further information do you need?

FINDINGS

Uterine contractions are infrequent and seem to be getting farther apart. There are no other signs of labor and no leaking of amniotic fluid.

ANALYSIS

Labor does not seem to be occurring. Yolanda needs to continue to watch for signs of labor, infection, bleeding, and leaking of amniotic fluid.

ACTIONS

What counseling/teaching is needed now?

32. **Critical Thinking Challenge:** The following situation has been developed to challenge your critical thinking. Read the situation and then answer "yes" or "no" to the question that follows.

Your client, Amy Lightfoot, is a 15-year-old gravida 1 who is in her 35th week of pregnancy with severe preeclampsia. An amniocentesis is done to assess fetal lung maturity. Test results indicate an L/S ratio of 2:1 and that prostaglandin (PG) is present.

Is Fetal Lung Maturity Indicated?

Yes _____   No _____

Explain your answer:

33. **Memory Check:** Define the following abbreviations.

    a. AFI   j. IUGR

    b. BSST   k. L/S ratio

    c. BPP   l. MSAFP

    d. CRL   m. NST

    e. CST   n. ntt

    f. CVS   o. PG

    g. FHR   p. US

    h. FL   q. VAS

    i. HC

CHAPTER 11

PROCESSES AND STAGES OF LABOR AND BIRTH

Successful labor and birth result from the effective interplay of five critical factors. This chapter considers the role of each of these factors in the process of birth. This chapter corresponds to Chapter 22 in the eighth edition of *Olds' Maternal-Newborn Nursing & Women's Health Across the Lifespan.*

BIRTH PASSAGE

1. *Critical factors in labor:* Two of the five critical factors in labor are the birth passage and psychosocial considerations.

   a. Explain why the birth passage is considered a critical factor.

   b. Explain why psychosocial considerations are a critical factor.

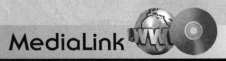

MediaLink

http://www.prenhall.com/davidson

Additional resources for this content can be found on the Student DVD-ROM accompanying the eighth edition of *Olds' Maternal-Newborn Nursing & Women's Health Across the Lifespan,* and on the Companion Website at http://www.prenhall.com/davidson. Click on the text chapter number(s) listed for this content to select the appropriate activities.

Prentice Hall Nursing MediaLink DVD-ROM
- Audio Glossary
- NCLEX Review

Companion Website
- Additional NCLEX Review
- Case Study: Client in First Stage Labor
- Care Plan Activity: Client in Second Stage of Uncomplicated Labor
- Care Plan Activity: Identifying Appropriate Labor Progress

2. The majority of women have a gynecoid pelvis. The anthropoid pelvis is the second most common pelvic type. What characteristics of these pelves make them advantageous for birth?

3. The android and platypelloid pelves are unfavorable for vaginal birth. What unfavorable characteristics are present in each type?

4. Draw the shape of the pelvic inlet for each type of pelvis and mark the favorable characteristics with red pen to make them stand out.

5. The anterior-posterior diameter of the pelvic inlet is estimated from manual measurement of the

   a. obstetric conjugate.

   b. diagonal conjugate.

   c. conjugate vera.

   d. intertuberishii.

6. The normal anterior-posterior diameter of the inlet needs to be at least

   a. 8 cm.

   b. 9 cm.

   c. 10 cm.

   d. 11 cm.

THE FETUS

7. Label the parts of the fetal skull indicated in Figure11–1.

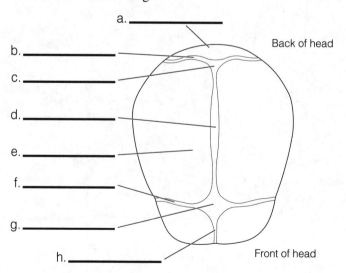

Figure 11–1 Superior view of the fetal skull.

8. Define *suture*.

Match the type of suture with its location.

9. _____ Coronal suture

10. _____ Mitotic (frontal) suture

11. _____ Sagittal suture

12. _____ Lambdoidal suture

   a. Between the parietal bones and the occipital bone

   b. Between the parietal bones and the frontal bones

   c. Between the frontal bones

   d. Between the parietal bones

13. Define *fontanelle*. Why are fontanelles important in the fetal skull?

14. Describe the location and characteristic size of the following:

   a. Anterior fontanelle

   b. Posterior fontanelle

15. Label the landmarks of the fetal skull indicated on Figure11–2.

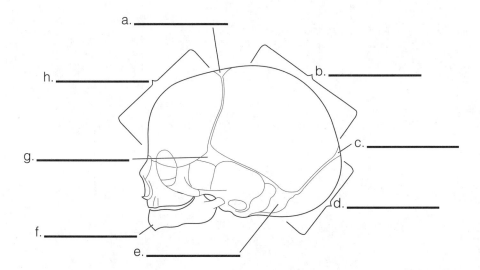

Figure 11–2   Lateral view of the fetal skull identifying the landmarks that have significance during birth.

16. Figure 11–3 depicts the anteroposterior and transverse diameters of the fetal head. Label each of the diameters and state the "norms" for an average size full-term newborn.

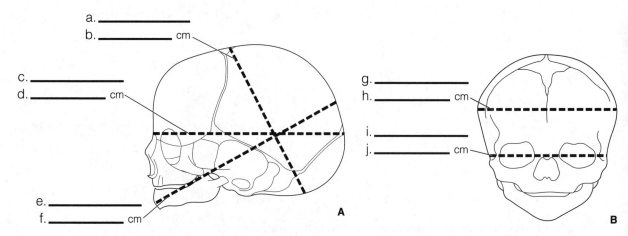

a. _____
b. _____ cm
c. _____
d. _____ cm
e. _____
f. _____ cm

g. _____
h. _____ cm
i. _____
j. _____ cm

A

B

Figure 11–3 *A,* Anteroposterior diameters of the fetal skull when the vertex of the fetus presents and the fetal head is flexed with the chin on the chest; the smallest anteroposterior diameter (suboccipitobregmatic diameter) enters the birth canal. *B,* Transverse diameters of the fetal skull.

Match the following terms with the correct definitions.

17. _____ Fetal position

18. _____ Fetal attitude

19. _____ Fetal lie

a. Relationship of the cephalocaudal axis of the fetus to the cephalocaudal axis of the woman

b. Relationship of the landmark on the presenting fetal part to the anterior, posterior, or sides of the maternal pelvis

c. Relationship of the fetal parts to one another

20. Draw a fetus in a longitudinal lie and a transverse lie on Figure 11–4.

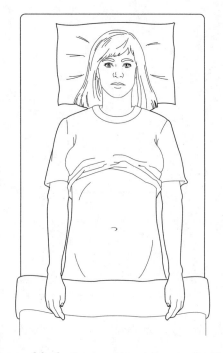

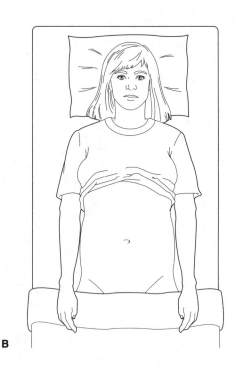

A

B

Figure 11–4 Fetal position. *A,* Longitudinal lie *B,* Transverse lie.

21. Define *fetal presentation*.

22. List the four types of cephalic presentation.

   a.   c.

   b.   d.

23. List and describe the three types of breech presentation. Explain how they are different.

   a.

   b.

   c.

Label the fetal presentations and positions shown in Figure 11–5.

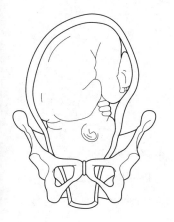 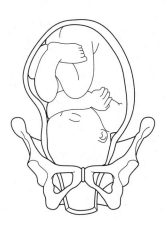 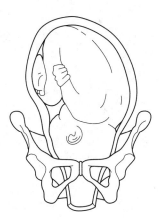

24. a. presentation _____   25.   a. presentation _____   26.   a. presentation _____

      b. position _____   b. position _____   b. position _____

      c. presenting part _____   c. presenting part _____   c. presenting part _____

Figure 11–5 Categories of presentation.

SOURCE: Courtesy Ross Laboratories, Columbus, OH.

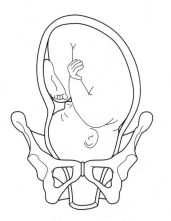

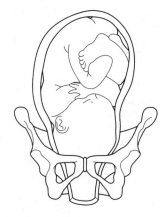

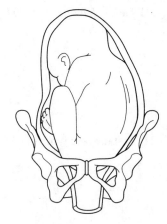

27. a. presentation _____
    b. position _____
    c. presenting part _____

28. a. presentation _____
    b. position _____
    c. presenting part _____

29. a. presentation _____
    b. position _____
    c. presenting part _____

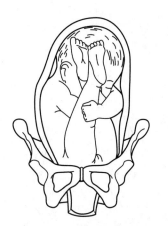

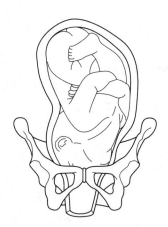

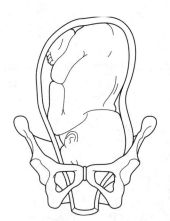

30. a. presentation _____
    b. position _____
    c. presenting part _____

31. a. presentation _____
    b. position _____
    c. presenting part _____

32. a. presentation _____
    b. position _____
    c. presenting part _____

Figure 11–5   Categories of presentation. (*continued*)
SOURCE: Courtesy Ross Laboratories, Columbus, OH.

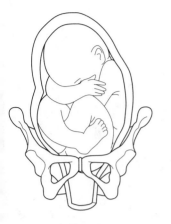

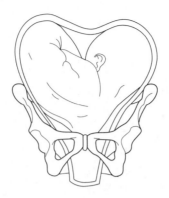

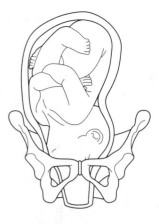

33. a. presentation _____

    b. position _____

    c. presenting part _____

34. a. presentation _____

    b. position _____

    c. presenting part _____

35. a. presentation _____

    b. position _____

    c. presenting part _____

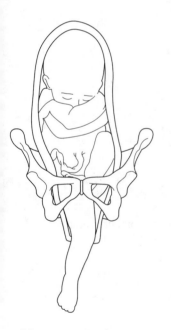

36. a. presentation _____

    b. position _____

    c. presenting part _____

Figure 11–5 Categories of presentation. (*continued*)
SOURCE: Courtesy Ross Laboratories, Columbus, OH.

37. List three methods that could be used to determine presentation and position.

    a.

    b.

    c.

38. Define *engagement.*

39. What information does engagement provide about adequacy of the inlet, midpelvis, and outlet?

40. Describe two methods used to determine engagement.

    a.

    b.

41. Devise two questions you could ask the expectant mother that would elicit information about symptoms indicative of engagement. Include your rationale.

    a.

    b.

42. Define *station.* How is station assessed?

43. Explain what a–1 station is.

44. Explain why the fetal presentation part may not descend.

UTERINE CONTRACTIONS

Match the term on the left to the correct definition on the right.

45. _____ Acme   a. The building up of the contraction

46. _____ Decrement   b. The letting up of the contraction

47. _____ Duration   c. The peak of the contraction

48. _____ Frequency   d. From the beginning of one to the beginning of the next contraction

49. _____ Increment   e. The time from the beginning to the end of one contraction

50. _____ Intensity   f. The strength of the contraction

51. Label each of the areas indicated in Figure 11–6.

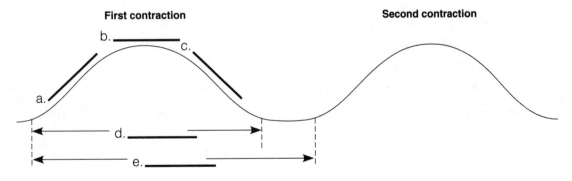

Figure 11–6   Characteristics of uterine contractions.

PSYCHOSOCIAL-CULTURAL CONSIDERATIONS

52. Amy Potts is 18 years old and in early labor. Identify the factors that may affect Amy's psychologic response to labor.

53. Describe how a woman's cultural background and preparation for labor might affect her psychologic status in labor.

PHYSIOLOGY OF LABOR

54. Which of the following are considered premonitory signs of labor?

    a. Bloody show, desire to bear down

    b. Desire to bear down, increased vaginal secretions

    c. Lightening, increased vaginal secretions

    d. Rupture of membranes, elevated temperature

55. There are various theories regarding the cause of labor onset. One possible cause involves

    a. an increase in the amount of circulating progesterone.

    b. a decrease in the amount of circulating estrogen.

    c. inactivation of phospholipase A_2.

    d. production of endogenous oxytocin by the mother's pituitary gland.

56. The fetus adapts to the birth canal by undergoing some positional changes. Which of the following answers best describes the correct sequence?

    a. Descent and flexion, extension, internal rotation, external rotation

    b. Extension, descent and flexion, internal rotation, external rotation

    c. Internal rotation, descent and flexion, extension, external rotation

    d. Descent and flexion, internal rotation, extension, external rotation

57. Labor and birth are divided into four stages, each with a definite beginning and ending. Complete the following chart:

Stage	Begins	Ends
First		
Second		
Third		
Fourth		

58. The first stage of labor is divided into which three phases?

    a.

    b.

    c.

Case Study: Read the following scenario, then answer questions 59–61.

Sally Reed, a primigravida, is admitted to the birthing center. Sally states that she has been having contractions for 4 hours and her water broke just a little while ago. She is excited that she is in labor. An admission assessment reveals that the fetal heart rate is 140; the contraction frequency is every 4–5 minutes, duration 40 seconds, intensity mild to moderate. Her cervix is 3 cm dilated and 50% effaced; fetal presentation is vertex, fetal station is –2, and the Nitrazine test tape is positive for amniotic fluid.

59. What stage and phase of labor is Sally in?

60. a. How much dilatation would you expect every hour for Sally?

    b. How would this be different if Sally were a multigravida?

61. What will contractions probably be like when Sally is in the active phase?

REFLECTIONS

Frequently the experience of labor is much different from the "norms" that textbooks address because each individual is different. What was your labor or the labor of a client like? Did it match the characteristics that you are learning about now? How was it different?

_____

_____

_____

_____

_____

62. Discuss the physiologic causes of pain during labor and birth.

63. Identify key factors that affect the woman's response to pain.

64. **Memory Check:** Define the following abbreviations (may have more than one answer).

   a. LADA   d. LMP

   b. LADP   e. LMT

   c. LMA   f. LOA

g. LOP

h. LOT

i. LSA

j. LSP

k. LST

l. RMA

m. RMP

n. RMT

o. ROA

p. ROM

q. ROP

r. ROT

s. RSA

t. RSP

u. RST

v. SROM

w. AROM

CHAPTER 12

NURSING ASSESSMENT AND CARE OF THE INTRAPARTAL FAMILY

Today, the birthing nurse must have a thorough understanding of the stages and processes of labor and the ability to correlate that knowledge with observable behavior and changes in the laboring woman and those supporting her. In essence, the nurse's understanding of labor and birth forms the basis for ongoing assessment, intervention, and evaluation of care during labor and birth.

This chapter corresponds to Chapters 23, 24, 25, and 27 in the eighth edition of *Olds' Maternal-Newborn Nursing & Women's Health Across the Lifespan.*

INITIAL ASSESSMENT AND ADMISSION

1. The following questionnaire is similar to many that are used when a woman is admitted to the labor and birth unit. Have a friend or family member act as a client and role-play a situation in which you, as the labor and birth nurse, complete the interview. (Note: This questionnaire focuses primarily on baseline information and does not include information that would require physical assessment.)

MediaLink

http://www.prenhall.com/davidson

Additional resources for this content can be found on the Student DVD-ROM accompanying the eighth edition of *Olds' Maternal-Newborn Nursing & Women's Health Across the Lifespan,* and on the Companion Website at http://www.prenhall.com/davidson. Click on the text chapter number(s) listed for this content to select the appropriate activities.

Prentice Hall Nursing MediaLink DVD-ROM
- Audio Glossary
- NCLEX Review
- Animation Tutorial: Rupturing Membranes
- Video Tutorial: Normal Vaginal Delivery
- Animation Tutorial: Placental Delivery

Companion Website
- Additional NCLEX Review
- Case Study: Maternal Assessment During Labor
- Case Study: Labor and Birth
- Case Study: Pain Management During Labor
- Care Plan Activity: Client on Pitocin with Decelerations
- Care Plan Activity: Client with Extended Family in Uncomplicated Labor
- Care Plan Activity: Pain Management in a Laboring Woman

Admission date _____ Time _____

Admitting nurse _____

Client name _____ Age _____

EDB _____ LMP _____ Length of gestation

by dates _____

Attending MD/CNM _____

Pediatrician _____

Gravida _____ Para _____ PT _____ Ab _____ Living children _____

Onset of labor: Spontaneous _____ Induced _____ Time _____ Bleeding _____

Membrane status: Intact _____ Ruptured _____ Time _____

Blood type & Rh _____ Serology _____ Rubella titer _____ HbSAg _____

Persons for maternal support during birth _____

Prenatal education classes: Yes _____ No _____ Type _____

Birthing requests: Feeding method: Breast _____ Formula _____ Glucose water _____

Pacifier _____

Ambulation: Yes _____ No _____

Shower: Yes _____ No _____ Jacuzzi: Yes _____ No _____ Continuous fetal

monitor: Yes _____ No _____

Choices of labor position _____ Birthing position _____

Medication during labor: Yes _____ No _____ Regional block: Yes _____ No _____

Birth requests _____

Other _____

Prepregnancy weight _____ Present weight _____ Weight gain _____

Allergy: Medications _____ Foods _____ Substances _____

Time of last food intake _____ Type _____ Fluids _____

Medical problems before pregnancy _____

Problems with last pregnancy _____

Problems with this pregnancy _____

2. Ann Bailey is admitted to the birthing center accompanied by her husband Roy. She is in early labor. During your initial interview, you discover that she is a primigravida and that her expected date of birth (EDB) is today. She has not attended prenatal classes. What four observations will you make while assessing her contractions?

   a.

   b.

   c.

   d.

3. Why do you use your fingertips instead of the palm of your hand to palpate contractions?

4. What would you expect Ann's contractions to be like if she is in the latent phase?

5. The charge nurse records Ann's contractions as every 5 minutes, lasting 30 seconds, and of mild intensity.
   a. What is the frequency? _____
   b. What is the duration? _____
   c. What is the intensity? _____

6. Roy hands you a piece of paper with a recording of contractions before admission. The paper shows:

Contraction Begins	Contraction Ends
0500:00	0500:40
0505:00	0505:40
0508:00	0508:45
0511:00	0511:45

   a. What is the frequency of the contractions? _____
   b. What is the duration of the contractions? _____

7. What differences would you perceive when palpating mild, moderate, and strong (intense) contractions?

8. You will use a handheld Doppler to assess fetal heart rate (FHR).

    a. Describe the method you will use to locate the FHR.

    b. After locating the fetal heartbeat and just before counting the FHR, you check Ann's radial pulse. Explain the rationale for this.

    c. How long should you listen to the FHR? At what times will it be important to assess the FHR?

9. As part of your assessment, you perform Leopold's maneuvers on Ann. How should she be positioned?

10. When you do Leopold's maneuvers, you feel a firm, rounded object in the uterine fundus; a smooth surface along the right side of the uterus (mother's right side); a surface that feels more nodular on the left side of the uterus; and a body part that is rounded and even more firm just above the symphysis.

    a. The fetal presentation is _____.

    b. The fetal position is _____.

11. Explain why membrane status should be ascertained before a vaginal examination is done.

12. What effect do intact membranes have on labor progress?

13. Explain the implications of ruptured membranes for the mother and fetus.

14. Why do you need to know the exact time that the membranes rupture?

15. Explain why the FHR is assessed immediately after the membranes have ruptured.

16. Ann says she doesn't think she wants her membranes ruptured artificially, but she's not sure. She asks, "What do you think I should do?" Write out your answer. Remember, because you want to help her be an informed consumer, your answer needs to include assessment of Ann's knowledge and understanding, an overview of the purpose of amniotomy, advantages, disadvantages, and any known alternatives to the amniotomy.

17. To practice your role as client advocate, imagine you have just carefully explained an amniotomy to a woman, and she decides she doesn't want it done. The physician calls in and says, "I'm on my way to the birthing unit to see Mrs. X. I'm planning to do an amniotomy if all is going well." What will your response be?

18. While examining Mrs. X, the physician says, "Hand me an amniohook so I can rupture these membranes." Mrs. X quickly looks to you, shaking her head from side to side. What will you say?

19. Ann states that she is losing some clear fluid from her vagina when she coughs. You note that the Nitrazine test tape does not change color.

    a. Are the membranes intact or ruptured?

    b. What do you think the source of the clear fluid is?

20. You do a vaginal examination on Ann.

    a. List the information that can be ascertained by performing a vaginal examination.

    b. How do you position Ann for the vaginal examination? What will you do to protect her privacy?

21. When the physician attempts to perform a sterile vaginal examination, Ann becomes extremely anxious and is tearful.

    a. What factors could contribute to Ann's response?

    b. Describe what you would say to Ann to decrease her anxiety and fear and make the examination more comfortable.

22. During the vaginal examination, you find that you can place two fingers side by side in Ann's cervix. You can feel a firm surface against the cervix and a softer triangular shape in the upper right position (between 12 and 3 on a clock). You also note a small amount of bloody show.

    a. What is the cervical dilatation?

    b. What is the presentation?

    c. What is the position?

    d. What causes the bloody show?

BREATHING TECHNIQUES

23. Choose a breathing technique commonly used in your area. Now, select a friend and teach her or him the breathing pattern you chose. Write out a description or draw the breathing pattern so you will be ready for your clinical experience.

24. What can you do to help Roy during the birth process? How can you assist him in supporting Ann? Describe support and comfort measures you can teach him or that you can provide if needed.

FETAL MONITORING

The physician has recommended fetal monitoring for a short time. After the reason for it is explained, Ann agrees to having a monitor placed on her abdomen.

25. Define the following terms used with fetal monitoring:

   a. Fetal baseline

   b. Fetal tachycardia

   c. Fetal bradycardia

   d. Baseline variability

   e. Early deceleration

   f. Late deceleration

   g. Variable deceleration

26. Spell out the following abbreviations used in fetal monitoring:

    a. EFM

    b. FHR

    c. UA

27. The normal fetal heart rate is (a) _____ to (b) _____ beats per minute, baseline variability is (c) _____, there are accelerations with fetal movement, and there are (d) _____ late or variable decelerations.

28. List three possible causes of fetal tachycardia.

    a.

    b.

    c.

29. List three possible causes of fetal bradycardia.

    a.

    b.

    c.

30. While you are caring for a woman in labor, you notice the fetal heart rate drop to the 90 range for 2 minutes. What do you do?

31. List three possible causes of changes in baseline variability.

    a.

    b.

    c.

32. Explain the causes and the physiologic rationale for the following:

    a. Early deceleration

    b. Late deceleration

    c. Variable deceleration

33. Evaluate the fetal monitoring strip shown in Figure 12–1.

    a. Contraction frequency _____

    b. Contraction duration _____

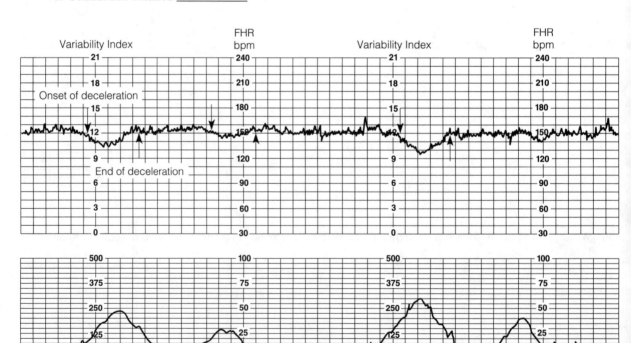

Figure 12–1 Evaluation of EFM tracing.

c. Type of FHR pattern (check one of the following):

_____ no decelerations

_____ early decelerations

_____ late decelerations

_____ variable decelerations

d. Circle each deceleration you find.

34. Evaluate the fetal monitoring strip shown in Figure 12–2.

a. Contraction frequency _____

b. Contraction duration _____

c. Type of FHR pattern (check one of the following):

_____ no decelerations   _____ late decelerations

_____ early decelerations   _____ variable decelerations

d. Variability (check one of the following):

_____ marked   _____ average   _____ minimal

e. Is contraction frequency within normal expectations?

_____ yes _____ no

f. Is contraction duration within normal expectations?

_____ yes _____ no

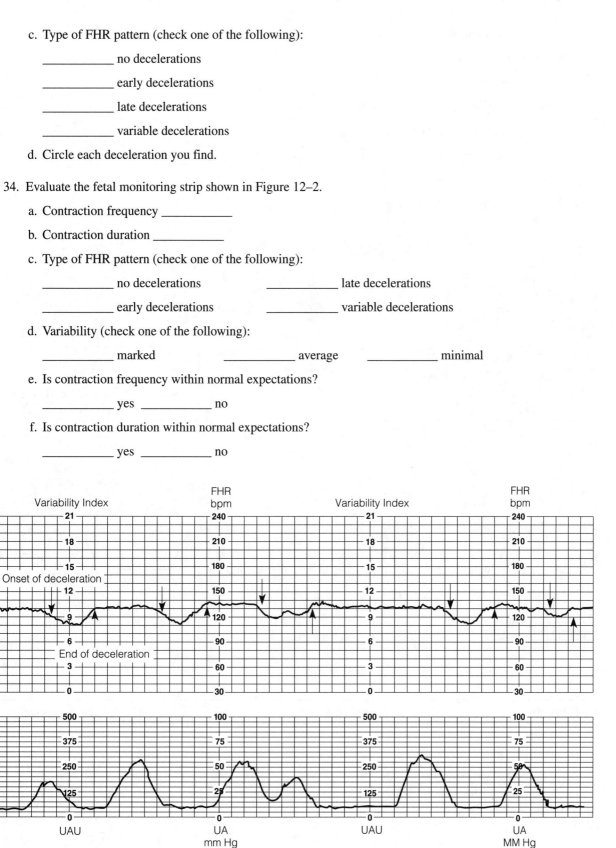

Figure 12–2   Evaluation of EFM tracing.

35. Evaluate the fetal monitoring strip shown in Figure 12–3.

    a. Contraction frequency _____

    b. Contraction duration _____

    c. Type of FHR pattern (check one of the following):

       _____ early decelerations

       _____ late decelerations

       _____ variable decelerations

    d. Circle each deceleration you find.

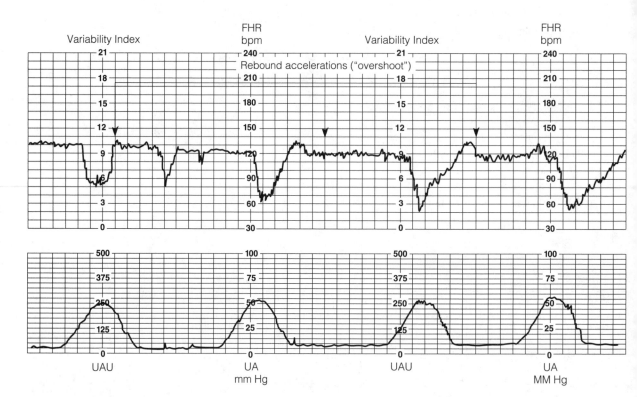

Figure 12–3 Evaluation of EFM tracing.

36. Identify the immediate nursing actions and physiologic rationale for the following FHR problems:

FHR Problem	Nursing Actions	Physiologic Rationale
Late decelerations		
Variable decelerations		

37. The fetal heart rate assessment by EFM has indicated a normal pattern. At 5 to 6 cm dilatation, Ann asks for a pain medication. Stadol 1 mg IVP is ordered and is to be given by the RN in the birthing unit.

    a. Describe the assessments needed before administering the medication.

    b. Describe assessments to be made after administering the medication.

    c. List at least two indications that the medication is exerting the expected effect.

38. Ann reaches 8 cm and becomes restless and impatient. What phase of labor is she in?

ASSESSMENT AND SUPPORT DURING LABOR

39. Ann begins to indicate many signs of discomfort and anxiety. Her previous methods to increase relaxation are no longer effective. Based on your assessment, you select the nursing diagnosis *Acute Pain related to anxiety and difficulty maintaining relaxation.* Identify at least four nursing interventions you think are important. Explain the physiologic rationale for each intervention.

    a. **Nursing Intervention**   **Physiologic Rationale**

    b. Identify two anticipated outcomes or two signs that would indicate your interventions have been effective.

40. Ann complains of tingling and numbness in her hands and feet.

    a. What is the cause?

    b. List nursing interventions to assist Ann.

    c. Identify findings that indicate your interventions have been effective.

41. Ann reaches complete dilatation.

    a. Complete dilatation is _____ cm.

    b. What stage of labor is Ann in?

42. List signs that indicate birth is imminent.

43. You prepare the birthing room for the birth. Describe the maternal positions that may be used during labor and birth. Identify the advantages and disadvantages of each, and determine one situation in which you might suggest the use of that particular position.

44. How often will you assess blood pressure and FHR in the second stage?

45. Explain the support and comfort measures you or Roy can use to help Ann feel more comfortable as birth approaches.

EPISIOTOMY

46. The physician tells Ann that an episiotomy is needed. Describe indications for an episiotomy.

47. In Figure 12–4, draw a midline, left mediolateral, and right mediolateral episiotomy.

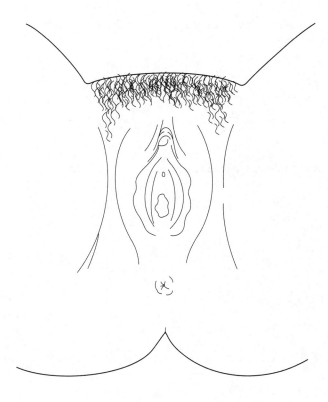

Figure 12–4

48. Complete the following chart regarding differences between a midline episiotomy and a mediolateral episiotomy.

Characteristic	Midline Episiotomy	Mediolateral Episiotomy
Indication		
Healing		
Discomfort after birth		

49. Discuss prenatal, labor, and birth measures and interventions that may decrease the need for an episiotomy.

BIRTH

50. As the baby's head begins to emerge, the obstetrician or certified nurse-midwife supports it with her or his hand. Explain the rationale for this.

51. Why are the baby's nose and mouth suctioned as soon as the head has emerged?

APGAR SCORE

52. A baby boy is born. Your first assessment of him provides the following information:

    Heart rate 124

    Respirations 24 and irregular

    Flexion and movement of all extremities

    Vigorous crying when suctioned with the bulb syringe

    Pink body with some acrocyanosis

    a. Record the preceding assessments on the Apgar scoring sheet (Figure 12–5).

    b. What is the total Apgar score? _____

    c. Apgar scores are assessed at _____ minutes and _____ minutes following birth.

	0	1	2
Heart rate	Absent	Slow (below 100)	Above 100
Respiratory effort	Absent	Slow, irregular	Good crying
Muscle tone	Flaccid	Some flexion of extremities	Active motion
Reflex irritability	None	Grimace	Vigorous cry
Color	Pale, blue	Body pink, extremities blue	Completely pink

Figure 12–5 Sample Apgar scoring sheet.

SOURCE: Modified from Apgar, V. (1966). The newborn [Apgar] scoring system: Reflection and advice. Pediatric Clinics of North America, 13, 645.

53. The most crucial of the Apgar assessments are the heart rate and respiration. If the baby has a pink body, what do you know about the baby's heartbeat and respiration?

NURSING CARE FOLLOWING BIRTH

54. List the methods that may be used to provide warmth to the newborn in the birthing room.

55. Why should the newborn be dried thoroughly as soon after birth as possible?

56. Ann places her newborn on her chest with skin-to-skin contact to maintain warmth. In some birth settings the newborn may be placed under a radiant heater. Explain how the radiant heater works.

57. As the nurse, you assess the number of vessels in the umbilical cord.

    a. Why is this important?

    b. How many vessels should there be?

58. List two methods of ensuring correct identification of the newborn after birth.

    a.

    b.

59. What positions may the baby be placed in to facilitate drainage of the respiratory tract?

60. What complication may result from vigorous, frequent oral suctioning?

61. List the areas that will be checked during a brief physical assessment of the newborn in the first few minutes after birth.

62. Describe ways in which you can facilitate attachment immediately after birth.

63. List specific maternal behaviors that would indicate Ann is beginning to establish attachment.

EXPULSION OF THE PLACENTA

64. List four signs that indicate separation of the placenta.

    a.

    b.

    c.

    d.

65. Describe differences between a Schultze and a Duncan expulsion of the placenta.

    a. Method of separation from the uterine wall

    b. Appearance of placenta at the moment of exit from the vagina

66. Ann's baby was born 20 minutes ago and the placenta still has not been expelled. Ann asks if this is normal. What do you tell her?

67. List three assessments of the expelled placenta that need to be made.

NURSING CARE IN THE THIRD STAGE

68. The obstetrician orders 10 units of Pitocin added to the IV solution after expulsion of the placenta.

    a. Explain the rationale for administration of an oxytocic medication following expulsion of the placenta.

    b. Identify the most important nursing interventions when administering Pitocin.

69. You need to record the length of each stage on Ann's birth record, based on the following information:

    Contractions began at 0800

    Complete dilatation at 1600

    Male infant born at 1710

    Placenta expelled at 1725

    a. First stage _____

    b. Second stage _____

    c. Third stage _____

    d. Fourth stage _____

70. How does the length of each of Ann's stages compare with "norms" for primigravidas?

NURSING CARE IN THE FOURTH STAGE

Ann begins her recovery period after birth. For each of the critical nursing assessments listed, indicate the expected normal findings. Circle the correct answer.

71. Blood pressure and pulse

    a. at prepregnant level

    b. elevated

    c. same as in labor

72. Uterine fundus height

    a. above umbilicus

    b. at umbilicus

    c. below umbilicus

73. Uterine fundus—position

    a. midline

    b. to maternal left

    c. to maternal right

74. Uterine fundus—consistency

    a. firm

    b. soft

    c. not able to locate

75. Lochia—amount

    a. heavy

    b. moderate

    c. scant

76. Lochia—color

    a. alba

    b. rubra

    c. serosa

77. Lochia—presence of clots

    a. baseball size

    b. golf ball size

    c. none

78. Perineum—episiotomy

    a. suture intact

    b. some gaping of sutures

79. Perineum—bruising

    a. marked ecchymosis

    b. none to minimal

80. Perineal—swelling

    a. marked

    b. none or slight

81. Bladder distention

    a. distended

    b. nondistended

82. What is the significance of a boggy uterus? Describe the immediate action you would take if the uterus were boggy.

83. Ann complains of episiotomy discomfort. List some measures that may alleviate her discomfort.

84. The recovery period usually extends for 1 to 2 hours after birth. List criteria that suggest normal recovery and that indicate the frequent assessments may cease.

PAIN DURING LABOR: CONTRIBUTING FACTORS, SUPPORT, ANALGESICS, AND ANESTHETICS

85. List the physiologic factors that contribute to discomfort in each stage of labor.

    a. First stage

    b. Second stage

    c. Third stage

86. How do each of the following factors influence the perception of pain in the laboring woman?

    a. Cultural background

    b. Fatigue

    c. Anxiety

    d. Previous experience

87. The nurse completes pertinent assessments of the mother, the baby, and the labor before administering analgesics during labor. For each of the following, indicate findings that should be present before administration of the analgesic.

    a. Maternal assessment

    b. Fetal assessment

    c. Labor assessment

88. Queen Jones, gravida 1, para 0, is in the active phase of labor. Contractions are every 3 minutes, last 50 seconds, and are moderate. She is 4 cm dilated, 75% effaced, and at 0 station. Her membranes are intact, and the FHR is 140. With each contraction, Queen cries out and thrashes in the bed. Her restlessness continues between contractions. She repeatedly changes positions and rolls her head from side to side. Her blood pressure and pulse rate have increased over the past 2 hours. The physician has ordered 75 mg of meperidine (Demerol) and 25 mg of promethazine given intramuscularly when needed for pain.

    a. In the preceding statement, circle all the findings that indicate it would be safe to administer the ordered medication. (Note: See answer to question 87 to assist you if you are having difficulty.)

    b. Identify the three most important nursing considerations regarding administration of medication.

    c. If all you have is a 100 mg/1 mL ampule of Demerol, how much will you draw up in your syringe?

    d. Identify the landmarks you would use to administer the medication in the

       (1) dorsogluteal site.

       (2) ventrogluteal site.

89. If Queen continues to experience discomfort and needs additional pain relief, what types of regional anesthesia might be given?

   a. In active labor:

   b. In second-stage labor:

REFLECTIONS

Describe the first birth that you were able to attend as a student nurse. What support measures were used? Did the expectant woman have a support person? How was the newborn welcomed into the world by those present? What were your feelings?

_____

_____

_____

_____

_____

_____

_____

_____

_____

_____

_____

_____

_____

90. Kim Ng, a 21-year-old gravida 1, para 0, is currently 2 cm dilated, with irregular contractions every 4 to 9 minutes, lasting 30 seconds and of mild intensity. She states she is in pain and would like an epidural. What do you do?

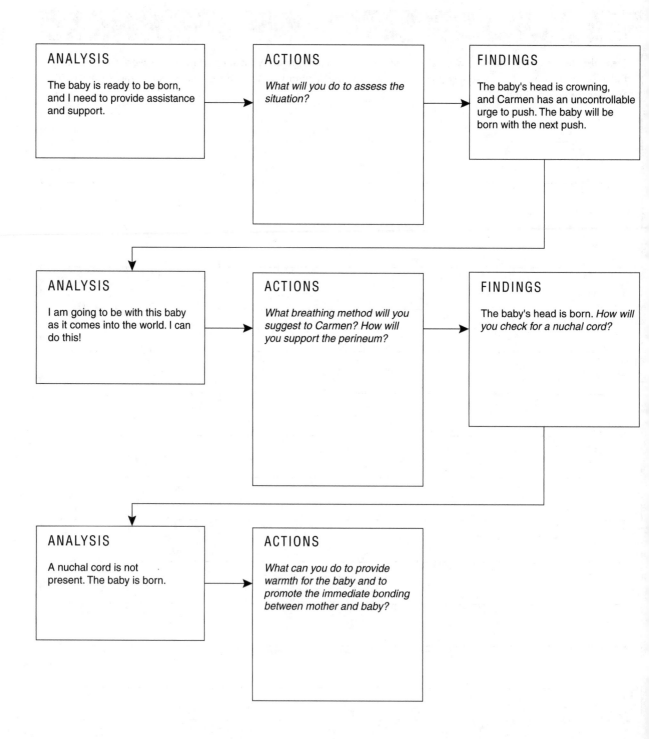

ANALYSIS

The baby is ready to be born, and I need to provide assistance and support.

ACTIONS

What will you do to assess the situation?

FINDINGS

The baby's head is crowning, and Carmen has an uncontrollable urge to push. The baby will be born with the next push.

ANALYSIS

I am going to be with this baby as it comes into the world. I can do this!

ACTIONS

What breathing method will you suggest to Carmen? How will you support the perineum?

FINDINGS

The baby's head is born. *How will you check for a nuchal cord?*

ANALYSIS

A nuchal cord is not present. The baby is born.

ACTIONS

What can you do to provide warmth for the baby and to promote the immediate bonding between mother and baby?

91. **Critical Thinking in Practice:** The following action sequence is designed to help you think through clinical problems. Read the following sequence, then fill in the appropriate boxes in the flowchart.

    You are the nurse in the birthing area. Carmen Lopez, a 25-year-old gravida 2, para 1, has been laboring for the past 6 hours. Suddenly you hear a low groan from her room, and then Carmen begins to shout, "The baby is coming!" You rush to her room.

92. **Memory Check:** Define the following abbreviations.

    a. Ab

    b. EDB

    c. EFM

    d. D & C

    e. epis

    f. FHR

    g. HC

    h. LMP

    i. Rh

    j. ROM

    k. VBAC

CHAPTER 13

CHILDBIRTH AT RISK

As her pregnancy advances, each woman wonders about the course of her labor and birth. Relatively smooth labor and birth of a healthy baby are, of course, the desired outcomes and are the result in the majority of cases. However, in some instances problems develop that complicate the process of birth and jeopardize the well-being of mother or baby, or both.

This chapter focuses on the complications that may arise during labor and birth. This chapter corresponds to Chapters 26, 27, and 37 in the eighth edition of *Olds' Maternal-Newborn Nursing & Women's Health Across the Lifespan.*

ANXIETY, FEAR, AND PSYCHOLOGIC DISORDERS

1. Anxiety affects the laboring woman and her baby. Explain the possible effects of increased anxiety and fear on the birth process.

2. Describe the signs and symptoms you might observe when a woman is experiencing depression.

MediaLink

http://www.prenhall.com/davidson

Additional resources for this content can be found on the Student DVD-ROM accompanying the eighth edition of *Olds' Maternal-Newborn Nursing & Women's Health Across the Lifespan,* and on the Companion Website at http://www.prenhall.com/davidson. Click on the text chapter number(s) listed for this content to select the appropriate activities.

Prentice Hall Nursing MediaLink DVD-ROM
- Audio Glossary
- NCLEX Review
- Video Tutorial: Cesarean Delivery

Companion Website
- Additional NCLEX Review
- Case Study: Client with Placental Problems
- Case Study: Client Undergoing Labor Induction
- Care Plan Activity: Prevention of Cord Prolapse in Laboring Woman
- Care Plan Activity: Client with Pitocin for Labor Augmentation

3. Identify at least one nursing diagnosis that would be important in decreasing a woman's anxiety and fear.

FAILURE TO PROGRESS

4. Compare the effects of hypertonic and hypotonic labor on the woman and her baby.

5. What does the term *failure to progress* mean?

6. Define the term *active management of labor* (AMOL).

7. Discuss the possible treatment regimens for hypotonic labor and failure to progress.

PRECIPITOUS LABOR AND BIRTH

8. Define *precipitous labor.*

9. Discuss the medical treatment that may be suggested for subsequent births when a woman has had a precipitous labor and birth.

POSTTERM PREGNANCY

Latisha Brown, a 21-year-old primipara, is pregnant with her first child. Latisha's last menstrual period (LMP) was September 8.

10. Her expected date of birth (EDB) is:

11. On what date would her pregnancy become postterm?

12. Latisha does have a postterm pregnancy. Why will the fetus be at increased risk of having a variable deceleration pattern? What other problems may occur during labor and birth?

FETAL MALPOSITION

Match the fetal malposition on the left with the descriptions on the right. More than one description may be used for each fetal malposition.

13. _____ Occiput posterior position

14. _____ Face presentation

15. _____ Brow presentation

16. _____ Transverse lie

a. Largest anteroposterior of the fetal head presents to the maternal pelvis.

b. The shoulder or acromion process is the presenting part.

c. A cesarean birth must be done.

d. The laboring woman experiences severe backache.

e. Pelvic rocking may convert the OP to OA.

f. The anteroposterior diameter of the fetal head is small, but the baby is at great risk during vaginal birth.

g. If the mentum is posterior, a cesarean is the method of birth.

17. Label each type of breech and the position of each in Figure 13–1.

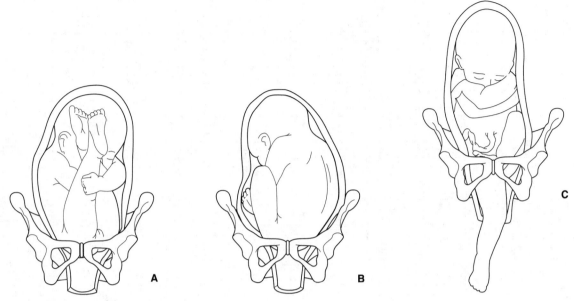

Figure 13–1 Types of breech.

a. _____   b. _____   c. _____

18. Breech presentation carries an increased risk of prolapse of the umbilical cord. Draw a prolapsed cord in Figure 13–1, *C*. Use a colored pen or pencil so it will stand out.

19. Prolapse of the cord causes pressure on the umbilical cord.

   a. Explain the fetal implications of a prolapsed cord.

   b. Describe what you would feel while performing a sterile vaginal examination, and what your immediate interventions must be.

   c. On Figure 13–2, draw the type of deceleration pattern that may occur with a prolapsed cord. First draw uterine contractions with a frequency of 3 minutes.

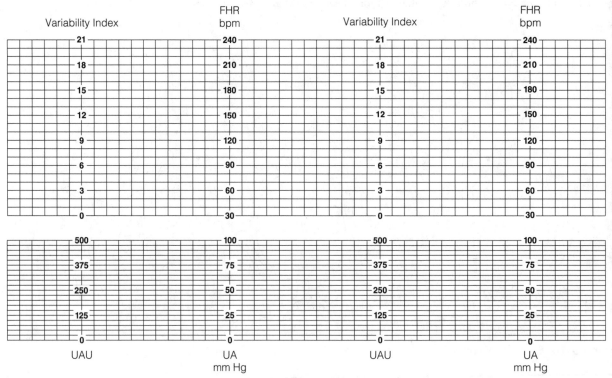

Figure 13–2 Fetal monitoring strip.

PLACENTAL PROBLEMS

20. Define *abruptio placentae*. What are the different types?

21. Define *placenta previa*. What are the different types?

Match the placental problems on the left with the descriptions on the right. Descriptions may be used more than once.

22. _____ Abruptio placentae (marginal)

23. _____ Abruptio placentae (central)

24. _____ Placenta previa (complete)

a. Bright-red bleeding without pain

b. Dark-red bleeding, may be associated with pain

c. Uterine tenderness and irritability

d. Normal uterine tone

e. Increased resting tone between contractions

f. Increased risk of DIC

25. Clare Sims is admitted at 38 weeks' gestation with abruptio placentae. She is at increased risk for DIC and HELLP. Why are these complications more likely to develop?

26. Rose Trujillo, gravida 3, para 1, is admitted with moderate vaginal bleeding. She is at 39 weeks' gestation. She states that she is not having contractions but that she has had episodes of vaginal bleeding since the 20th week. An ultrasound reading demonstrated a marginal placenta previa. The FHR is 140. You know that a vaginal examination is usually done on admission to assess cervical dilatation. Will you do a vaginal examination now? Give the rationale for your answer.

MACROSOMIA

27. Anita King-Davis is a 39-year-old gravida 2, para 1. Her last baby was born at 39 weeks and weighed 9 lb, 12 oz. Anita asks you what causes "large babies." Identify the risks for macrosomic infants.

28. What is the most significant intrapartum complication that can occur with macrosomia?

29. Identify three nursing diagnoses for Anita and her baby.

    a.

    b.

    c.

EXTERNAL CEPHALIC VERSION

30. At 38 weeks' gestation, an external version may be done to convert a breech presentation into a cephalic presentation.

    a. Identify the prerequisites for a version and include rationale.

    b. Discuss nursing interventions before, during, and after the version.

    c. Why would an Rh-negative woman need to receive Rh immune globulin (RhoGAM)?

    d. Write out the pertinent points you need to cover in discharge teaching.

INDUCTION OF LABOR

31. List two indications for induction of labor. Explain why the induction may need to be done.

    a.

    b.

32. Patricia Gomez is scheduled for induction of labor. She is at 40 weeks' gestation. Before induction, a CST is obtained and the results are positive. Identify any contraindications present in this example.

33. List additional factors that contraindicate induction.

TABLE 13–1 Prelabor status evaluation scoring (Bishop) system

	Assigned value			
Factor	**0**	**1**	**2**	**3**
Cervical dilatation	Closed	1–2 cm	3–4 cm	5 cm or more
Cervical effacement	0%–30%	40%–50%	60%–70%	80% or more
Fetal station	−3	−2	−1, 0	+1 or lower
Cervical consistency	Firm	Moderate	Soft	
Cervical position	Posterior	Midposition	Anterior	

Modified from Bishop, E. H. (1964). Pelvic scoring for elective induction. *Obstetrics & Gynecology, 24,* 266.

34. Explain the Bishop score (see Table 13–1). What implications would the following scores have on anticipated induction success?

   a. Score of 3

   b. Score of 9

35. Abby Clark is admitted for an induction. She is gravida 2, para 1, and at 42 weeks' gestation. Her membranes are intact. Amanda's obstetrician orders continuous fetal monitoring. After a 20-minute reactive baseline tracing an induction IV of 10 units of Pitocin in 1000 mL of 5% dextrose in lactated Ringer's is started. The Pitocin is to be started at 1 milliunit/min by IV infusion pump. How many milliliters per hour will be needed to infuse 1 milliunit/min?

36. Five-percent dextrose in water is not routinely used for Pitocin induction because of the risk of water intoxication. Describe the signs of water intoxication.

37. Describe the physical assessments and the findings that indicate Abby's infusion rate can be advanced.

38. Identify the problems that might occur in response to the Pitocin induction.

39. After the induction has been in process for 2 hours, you palpate strong contractions and note the following information on the fetal monitoring strip shown in Figure 13–3.

   a. FHR baseline is _____ beats per minute.

   b. Variability is present _____ absent _____.

   c. Variability is _____.

   d. Accelerations are present. Yes _____ No _____.

   e. Contraction frequency is _____.

   f. Contraction duration is _____.

   g. Based on your assessment, should the IV Pitocin infusion rate be advanced? Explain your decision.

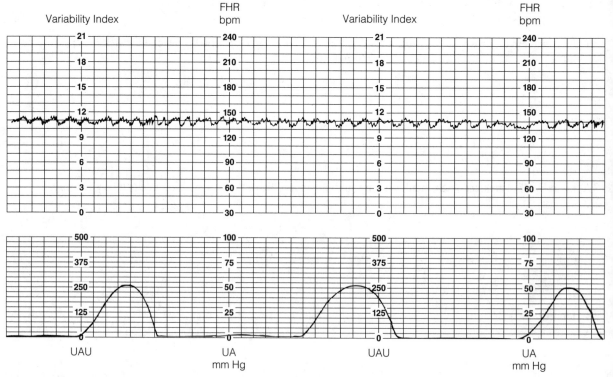

Figure 13–3   Fetal monitoring strip (6 small spaces equal 1 minute).

40. After an additional 1 hour of induction, you observe the fetal monitoring strip shown in Figure 13–4. What should you do?

a. What immediate nursing actions need to be taken?

b. What information from the strip did you use to determine your nursing actions?

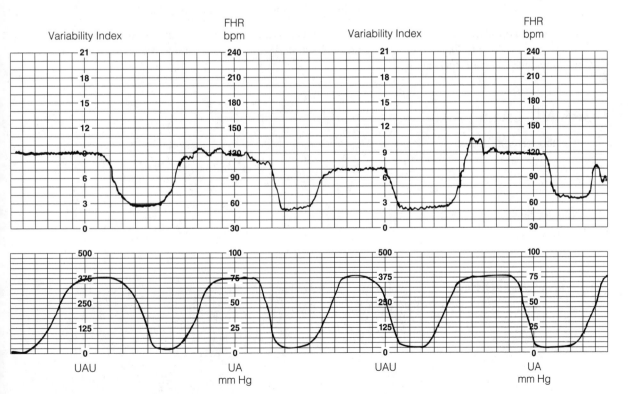

Figure 13–4   Fetal monitoring strip (6 small spaces equal 1 minute).

41. The obstetrician decides to rupture Abby's membranes.

    a. Why might this be done?

    b. What two assessments should be made immediately after the membranes are ruptured?

42. Explain the significance of the following characteristics of amniotic fluid:

    a. Greenish color

    b. Reddish color

    c. Foul odor

43. **Nursing Care Plan in Action:** For the following case scenario, focus on the pertinent data, formulate one appropriate nursing diagnosis, and complete all components of the nursing care plan.

    Case Scenario: Michelle, gravida 1, para 0, is admitted for induction because she has severe preeclampsia. In addition to IV Pitocin, she is receiving magnesium sulfate IV and O_2 at 7 L/min. Michelle's respirations are shallow with 10 breaths per minute.

NURSING CARE PLAN

Collaborative problems:

Nursing diagnosis:

Defining characteristics:

Goals: Client/husband will:		
Interventions	**Rationale**	**Expected Outcome**
Assessments:		
Nursing Interventions:		
Collaborative:		

44. Intravenous Pitocin may be used for augmentation of labor. Explain the differences between induction of labor and augmentation of labor.

45. Describe contraindications to augmentation.

46. If you note contraindications to the augmentation before beginning it, describe how you will communicate this information to the obstetrician.

47. Beth Ling is to be induced. A vaginal examination reveals 1 to 2 cm dilatation, 30% effacement, −2 station, cervical consistency moderate, and midposition.

   a. What is her Bishop Score?

   b. The physician decides to ripen the cervix. Describe the actions of dinoprostone (Cervidil or Prepidil).

   c. Beth's labor progresses and she receives an epidural. Discuss the key aspects of nursing care that will be required.

MULTIPLE PREGNANCY

48. Lydia Ruth is in her second pregnancy. List two signs and symptoms that may indicate the presence of twins.

   a.

   b.

49. Identify three complications that can occur with a multiple pregnancy.

   a.

   b.

   c.

50. Discuss the treatment that will be suggested for Lydia during her pregnancy.

51. Discuss the implications of the multiple pregnancy for the fetuses during labor and birth.

52. During labor, both fetuses will be monitored by electronic fetal monitoring. If one fetus begins to demonstrate problems with fetal heart rate (FHR), what will need to occur?

53. List three signs and symptoms that would indicate nonreassuring fetal status.

    a.

    b.

    c.

54. The major maternal complication that may occur following birth of twins is (a) _____.
    This occurs because (b) _____.

HYDRAMNIOS

55. Hydramnios occurs when there is more than _____ mL of amniotic fluid in the uterus.

56. Polly Brooks is diagnosed as having hydramnios. List three physical changes this may cause and identify at least two self-care measures you could suggest.

57. Identify three fetal problems associated with hydramnios and a method of identifying each problem.

    a.

    b.

    c.

58. When Polly's membranes rupture, she will be at increased risk for abruptio placentae. Explain the reason for this.

OLIGOHYDRAMNIOS

59. Define *oligohydramnios.*

60. Which fetal deceleration pattern are you more likely to see with oligohydramnios? Why?

61. Explain why oligohydramnios may be present when the fetus has a malformation or malfunction of the genitourinary system.

AMNIOINFUSION

62. Grace Yoo is also experiencing postterm pregnancy. Her CNM orders a biophysical profile to assess the fetus. The BPP is 6 with decreased amniotic fluid and a nonreactive nonstress test. The FHR exhibits numerous variable decelerations. The decision is made to treat the oligohydramnios and variable decelerations by inducing labor and then doing an amnioinfusion. What is an amnioinfusion and how do you know whether it is achieving the desired effect?

63. What other nursing intervention might you use to assist in relieving variable decelerations?

64. Why is the fetus at risk for meconium aspiration when oligohydramnios is present?

NONREASSURING FETAL STATUS: MECONIUM-STAINED AMNIOTIC FLUID

65. Pat Jones, gravida 3, para 2, is admitted with contractions every 2 minutes, lasting 60 seconds and of strong intensity. Her membranes ruptured spontaneously 2 hours ago, and Pat reports the fluid has been "greenish." She is breathing well with contractions and denies any discomfort. When assessing FHR, you located it above the umbilicus, at 140 beats per minute and regular. What would you suspect?

66. Explain the possible reasons for the presence of greenish amniotic fluid. What special measures will need to be taken for the newborn immediately after birth due to the presence of the green-stained fluid?

CEPHALOPELVIC DISPROPORTION

67. Mrs. Santos has a diagonal conjugate of 10 cm and converging side walls, and the fetal biparietal diameter (BPD) is 10 cm. What implications does this have for her labor and birth?

68. What types of evaluation methods would you expect to be done when cephalopelvic disproportion (CPD) is suspected?

69. Explain the rationale for a "trial of labor" (TOL) for a woman with borderline pelvic measurements.

70. What progress would you expect in cervical dilatation if the dilatation pattern remained within normal limits?

71. What progress would you expect in fetal descent?

72. In what instances would a cesarean need to be done?

73. Give an example in which the woman might need a cesarean for one birth and not for subsequent ones.

FORCEPS-ASSISTED BIRTH

74. List three indications for the use of forceps to assist in vaginal birth.

    a.

    b.

    c.

75. Identify the criteria that should be met in order for the obstetrician to use forceps safely.

76. Define the following:

    a. Outlet forceps

    b. Low forceps

    c. Mid-forceps

77. Identify complications (maternal and fetal) that may be associated with forceps.

78. Discuss the nursing interventions that are necessary during an outlet forceps–assisted birth. Include the teaching that should be done.

79. The new parents you worked with last evening during a forceps-assisted birth stop you in the hall today and ask why their baby's face is bruised and swollen on one side. They ask if it will go away. What will you tell them?

VACUUM EXTRACTOR–ASSISTED BIRTH

80. A vacuum extractor may be used instead of forceps.

   a. Explain how this works.

   b. Why might the baby have a "chignon"? Write out the important points to include in your parent teaching if the baby has a "chignon."

   c. Describe the teaching that will be needed before the use of the vacuum extractor. (Include maternal and fetal information.)

CESAREAN BIRTH

81. Kirsten Duncan, a 24-year-old gravida 2, para 1, at 36 weeks' gestation, is admitted to the birthing area for a repeat cesarean. Her primary (first) cesarean was done as an emergency measure when she began bleeding heavily from a complete placenta previa. The L/S ratio is 2.5:1 and PG is present.

   a. Describe how you will do the abdominal perineal prep.

   b. Describe the procedure for inserting an indwelling bladder catheter. What special implications does the low fetal head have on the insertion process?

   c. What teaching will you provide regarding the preoperative and postoperative course?

82. Kirsten's physician orders an IV. You insert an 18-gauge plastic cannula into the left forearm. The IV is to run at 150 mL/hr. The drop (gtt) factor is 15 gtt/mL. You will set the drip rate at _____ gtt/min.

83. Describe the location of the incision in the uterus of the following types of cesarean procedures:

    a. Low segment transverse

    b. Classic

84. List the advantages and disadvantages of a low segment transverse and classic uterine incision.

    a. Low segment transverse

    b. Classic

85. As a part of Kirsten's preoperative nursing care, you identified **Health-Seeking Behaviors related to lack of information about the postoperative course** as an important nursing diagnosis. You establish the nursing goal, "Provide information regarding the expected postoperative course" and select appropriate nursing interventions to accomplish this goal. Describe objective data that will show your teaching has been effective.

86. Describe the teaching you might do to help a father feel more comfortable during a cesarean birth.

VAGINAL BIRTH AFTER CESAREAN BIRTH (VBAC)

87. On her second postoperative day, Kirsten says to you, "If I have another baby, I would like to try to have a vaginal birth because she was so much smaller." What will you say?

REFLECTIONS

As you think about the clinical experiences you have had with childbearing women who were experiencing problems, what one woman or couple stands out in your mind? What were your feelings during that time? What type of problem was it? What was done to help? How did the situation turn out? How did the experience change you?

_____

_____

_____

_____

_____

_____

_____

_____

88. Becky Saunders asks if she could have a vaginal birth next time, even though she had a cesarean with her first birth.

   a. Which contraindications should be assessed?

   b. If she has a VBAC next time, she will be carefully assessed for which complications?

89. **Critical Thinking Challenge:** The following situation has been included to challenge your critical thinking. Read the situation and then select one answer on page 157.

   Carla James, a 22-year-old gravida 2, para 1, had a cesarean birth last time. She has a vertical incision on her abdomen and asks, "Does this mean that I can have a VBAC next time?"

Can Carla have a VBAC with her next birth?

Yes _____   Insufficient data _____   No _____

Explain your answer:

INTRAUTERINE FETAL DEATH

90. Anna Marner, a 19-year-old primipara at 33 weeks' gestation, calls the birthing unit and tells you she has not felt her baby move for 2 days.

    a. When she arrives, you admit her and listen for the FHR. You don't hear anything with the ultrasound Doppler. She says, "Did you hear my baby? Is she alive?" What will you say?

    b. What testing will you be able to anticipate for her?

91. Describe nursing care that will be important for Anna and her partner.

GRIEF

92. Nadine is a 36-year-old gravida 1, para 0 who conceived after 2 years of infertility. At 28 weeks, she experienced fluid leakage. She subsequently delivered a female fetus that appeared to have Down syndrome and subsequently died. What is the most appropriate response for you to say?

    a. "You wouldn't want to have a child with a birth defect anyway."

    b. "You can get pregnant again. If you conceived once, it'll happen again."

    c. "I'm very sorry for your loss."

    d. "I'll make sure to keep all visitors away so you can be alone."

93. The nurse calls Nadine 4 weeks later and Nadine states she feels very depressed and is constantly crying. What is your response?

94. **Memory Check:** Define the following abbreviations.

    a. AROM

    b. BPD

    c. CPD

    d. CS

    e. DIC

    f. HELLP

    g. IUFD

    h. mec st

    i. Pit

    j. SVE

    k. TOL

    l. VBAC

CHAPTER 14

NEWBORN PHYSIOLOGIC ADAPTATION AND ASSESSMENT

Today's neonatal nurse assesses neonatal development, identifies common variations in each newborn, and recognizes abnormalities. The nurse can then identify necessary early nursing interventions required for successful transition to home for the parent-infant unit.

This topic corresponds to Chapters 28 and 29 in the eighth edition of *Olds' Maternal-Newborn Nursing & Women's Health Across the Lifespan.*

PHYSIOLOGIC ADAPTATIONS

1. Describe four factors that are thought to stimulate the newborn to take his or her first breath.

   a.

   b.

   c.

   d.

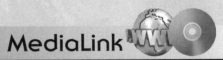

MediaLink

http://www.prenhall.com/davidson

Additional resources for this content can be found on the Student DVD-ROM accompanying the eighth edition of *Olds' Maternal-Newborn Nursing & Women's Health Across the Lifespan,* and on the Companion Website at http://www.prenhall.com/davidson. Click on the text chapter number(s) listed for this content to select the appropriate activities.

Prentice Hall Nursing MediaLink DVD-ROM
- Audio Glossary
- NCLEX Review
- Tools: Clinical Estimation of Gestational Age
- Tools: Maternal-Newborn Laboratory Values

Companion Website
- Case Study: Newborn Responses to Birth
- Additional NCLEX Review
- Case Study: Newborn Assessment
- Case Study: Newborn Maturity Assessment
- Care Plan Activity: Assessment of the Newborn
- Tools: Clinical Estimation of Gestational Age
- Tools: Maternal-Newborn Laboratory Values

2. State four anatomic and physiologic changes that occur in the cardiovascular system during the transition from fetal to neonatal circulation.

   a.

   b.

   c.

   d.

3. Newborn Zoe's temperature drops when she is placed on the cool plastic surface of the weight scales. This is an example of heat loss via

   a. conduction.

   b. convection.

   c. evaporation.

   d. radiation.

4. Describe the dialog you would use to teach a new mother about physiologic jaundice. Include why the time of onset of the jaundice is important.

REFLECTIONS

Do you remember the first time you held and cared for a newborn in your mother-baby rotation? How did you feel? What were your thoughts/impressions?

_____

_____

_____

_____

_____

_____

5. Discuss the expected level of development of the following senses in the newborn:

Sense	Assessment Method	Findings
Hearing		
Touch		
Taste/sucking		
Smell		

PERIOD OF REACTIVITY

6. Which time frame is most appropriate for the nursery nurse to initiate breastfeeding?

    a. The first period of reactivity.

    b. The first period of inactivity.

    c. The second period of inactivity.

    d. The second period of reactivity.

7. A primary nursing intervention appropriate to the second period of reactivity would be to

    a. auscultate the abdomen for the presence of bowel sounds.

    b. encourage the mother to begin breastfeeding.

    c. observe for excessive mucus.

    d. place infant under a radiant warmer.

8. Why is it important to determine the gestational age of all newborns?

GESTATIONAL AGE ASSESSMENT

As part of the admission process, the newborn's gestational age is determined. Using Ballard's gestational-age scoring tool (Figure 14–1 on page 163), determine Pam's gestational age based on the following assessments:

Pam's gestational physical exam yields the following assessments of her physical maturity: her skin is cracking and has a pale area; some areas have no lanugo present; the breast bud is 1 to 2 mm with stippled areola; the ears are formed and firm with instant recoil; plantar creases extend over anterior two thirds of sole; and the labia majora completely cover the minora and the clitoris. Assessment of Pam's neuromuscular development shows posture with flexion of the arms and hips, 0 degrees square window, 90 to 100 degrees arm recoil, popliteal angle of 110 degrees, scarf sign with elbow at midline, and a score of 4 for the head-to-ear maneuver.

9. Pam's Ballard score is (a)_____, which equates to a gestational age of

    (b) _____ weeks.

10. Pam's birth weight was 3202 g, her length was 49 cm, and her head circumference was 33.5 cm. Based on the gestational age you determined, correlate it with Pam's weight and classify her as LGA, AGA, or SGA. _____

    Plot Pam's length, weight, and head circumference on Figure 14–2 on page 164.

NEWBORN MATURITY RATING & CLASSIFICATION

ESTIMATION OF GESTATIONAL AGE BY MATURITY RATING
Symbols: X - 1st Exam O - 2nd Exam

NEUROMUSCULAR MATURITY

	−1	0	1	2	3	4	5
Posture							
Square Window (wrist)	>90°	90°	60°	45°	30°	0°	
Arm Recoil		180°	140°–180°	110°–140°	90°–110°	<90°	
Popliteal Angle	180°	160°	140°	120°	100°	90°	<90°
Scarf Sign							
Heel to Ear							

Gestation by Dates _____ wks

Birth Date _____ Hour _____ am / pm

APGAR _____ 1 min _____ 5 min

MATURITY RATING

score	weeks
−10	20
−5	22
0	24
5	26
10	28
15	30
20	32
25	34
30	36
35	38
40	40
45	42
50	44

PHYSICAL MATURITY

Skin	sticky friable transparent	gelatinous red, translucent	smooth pink, visible veins	superficial peeling &/or rash, few veins	cracking pale areas rare veins	parchment deep cracking no vessels	leathery cracked wrinkled
Lanugo	none	sparse	abundant	thinning	bald areas	mostly bald	
Plantar Surface	heel-toe 40–50 mm:−1 <40 mm:−2	>50 mm no crease	faint red marks	anterior transverse crease only	creases ant. 2/3	creases over entire sole	
Breast	imperceptible	barely perceptible	flat areola no bud	stippled areola 1–2 mm bud	raised areola 3–4 mm bud	full areola 5–10 mm bud	
Eye/Ear	lids fused loosely:−1 tightly:−2	lids open pinna flat stays folded	sl. curved pinna; soft; slow recoil	well-curved pinna; soft but ready recoil	formed & firm instant recoil	thick cartilage ear stiff	
Genitals male	scrotum flat, smooth	scrotum empty faint rugae	testes in upper canal rare rugae	testes decending few rugae	testes down good rugae	testes pendulous deep rugae	
Genitals female	clitoris prominent labia flat	prominent clitoris small labia minora	prominent clitoris enlarging minora	majora & minora equally prominent	majora large minora small	majora cover clitoris & minora	

Scoring system: Ballard, J.L., Khoury, J.C., Wedig K., Wang L., Eilers-Walsman, B.L., & Lipp, R. (1991). New Ballard Score, expanded to include extremely premature infants. *Journal of Pediatrics, 119*, 417–423.

SCORING SECTION

	1st Exam = X	2nd Exam = 0
Estimating Gest Age by Maturity Rating	_____Weeks	_____Weeks
Time of Exam	Date _____ Hour_____ am / pm	Date _____ Hour_____ am / pm
Age at Exam	_____ Hours	_____ Hours
Signature of Examiner	_____ M.D.	_____ M.D.

Figure 14–1   Newborn maturity rating & classification.

CLASSIFICATION OF NEWBORNS—
BASED ON MATURITY AND INTRAUTERINE GROWTH

Symbols: X-1st Exam O-2nd Exam

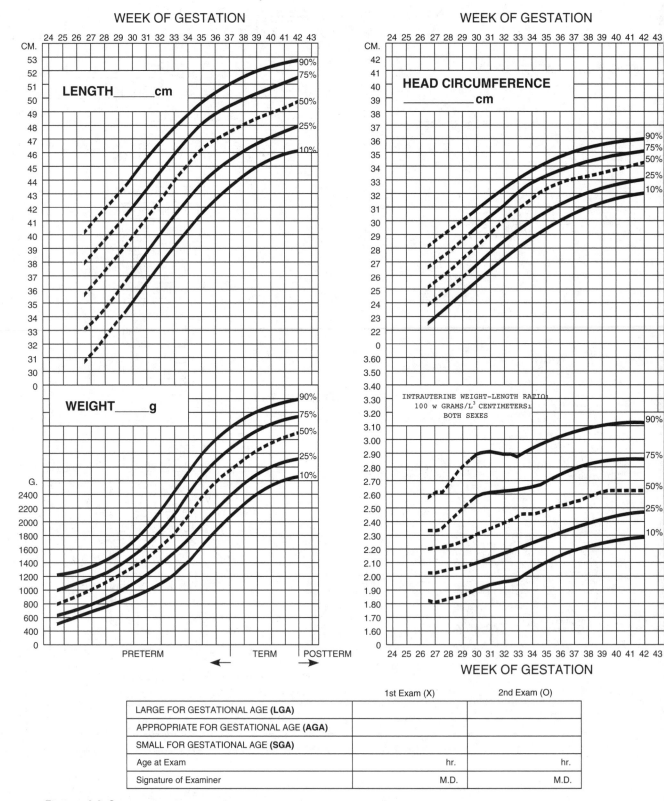

	1st Exam (X)	2nd Exam (O)
LARGE FOR GESTATIONAL AGE **(LGA)**		
APPROPRIATE FOR GESTATIONAL AGE **(AGA)**		
SMALL FOR GESTATIONAL AGE **(SGA)**		
Age at Exam	hr.	hr.
Signature of Examiner	M.D.	M.D.

Figure 14–2 Classification of newborns—based on maturity and intrauterine growth.

INITIAL ASSESSMENTS

11. List the normal range of values for the following newborn initial assessment areas:

Assessment Area	Normal Values
a. Temperature	
b. Pulse	
c. Respirations	
d. Blood pressure	

12. The average weight is (a) _____. Usual weight loss within the first 3 to 4 days of life for a full-term

    newborn is (b) _____%.

13. Why does the newborn commonly exhibit a "physiologic weight loss"?

14. A newborn's head circumference is 34 cm (13.6 in.) and chest circumference is 32 cm (12.5 in.). Which nursing action would be appropriate?

    a. Measure the occipitofrontal circumference daily.

    b. Prepare the mother for the probability that the healthcare provider will want to transilluminate the head.

    c. Record the findings and take no further action.

    d. Refer the newborn for evaluation for psychomotor delays.

15. Draw dotted lines on Figure 14–3 to show where you would measure a newborn's head and chest.

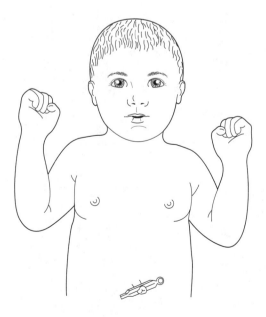

Figure 14–3   Measurement of newborn's head and chest.

16. Describe how you would accurately and safely measure the newborn's length.

17. Normal length range is _____.

18. The mother of a newborn questions the nurse about the rash on the neck and chest of her 24-hour-old newborn. The lesions are discrete, 2 mm, white papules on a pink base. What term would the nurse use to define this finding?

    a. Erythema toxicum

    b. Milia

    c. Mongolian spots

    d. Telangiectatic nevus (stork bites)

19. Which statement best defines a cephalhematoma?

    a. Diffuse edema of the scalp resulting from compression of local blood vessels

    b. Subperiosteal hemorrhage resulting from a traumatic birth

    c. Temporary reshaping of the skull resulting from the pressure of birth

20. On Figure 14–4, draw a series of numbered circles to indicate the correct sequence for auscultating a newborn's lungs. Place an "X" at the point where you should place your stethoscope in order to count the apical pulse.

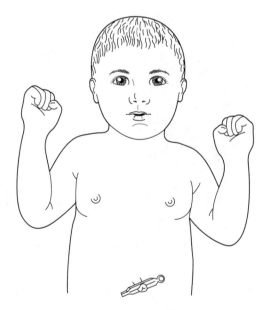

Figure 14–4   Auscultation of newborn's lungs and heart.

PHYSICAL ASSESSMENT OF THE NEWBORN

21. As the newborn nurse, you would complete an initial physical assessment of each newborn. Complete the following physical assessment chart.

Assessment Area	Normal Findings and Common Variations
Posture	
At rest	
Awake	
Skin	
Color	
Pigmentation	
Head	
Shape	
Sutures	
Fontanelles	
Face	
Eyes	
Position and Movement	
Conjunctiva	
Ears	
Placement	
Nose	
Patency	

(continued)

Assessment Area	Normal Findings and Common Variations
Mouth	
Gums	
Palate (hard and soft)	
Tongue	
Neck	
Clavicles	
Chest and Heart	
Shape	
PMI (Point of maximal intensity)	
Characteristics of pulses	
Lungs	
Characteristics of breath sounds	
Cry	
Abdomen	
Umbilical cord vessels	
Hips	
Extremities	
Position	
Movement	
Genitalia	

Assessment Area	Normal Findings and Common Variations
Spine	
Anus Placement and patency	
Neuromuscular Movement and tone	

22. While performing a newborn assessment, the nurse identifies the following when the bassinette is bumped: an extension of the arms, with fingers forming the shape of a "C." How would the nurse document this finding?

   a. Babinski's reflex

   b. Grasping reflex

   c. Moro reflex

   d. Tonic neck

23. The nurse tests the newborn's Babinski reflex by doing which of the following?

   a. Changing the newborn's equilibrium

   b. Placing a finger in the palm of the newborn's hand

   c. Stroking the lateral aspect of the sole from the heel upward and across the ball of the foot

   d. Touching the corner of the newborn's mouth or cheek

24. Identify three protective reflexes found in all normal newborns.

   a.

   b.

   c.

25. As you complete the newborn physical assessment, alteration in findings may be identified. Describe the defining physical characteristics or alterations and methods of assessment used for the following:

Hydrocephalus

Facial nerve palsy

Cleft palate

Omphalocele

Hypospadias

Myelomeningocele

Developmental dysplastic hip

Clubfoot

26. Why are the newborn's hands and feet often cold, and what is the term for the physical manifestation of this condition?

CHAPTER 15

NORMAL NEWBORN NEEDS AND CARE

The nurse identifies necessary nursing interventions, initial daily care needs including breastfeeding and formula feeding, and the discharge teaching required for successful transition to home for the parent-infant unit.

This chapter corresponds to Chapters 30 and 31 in the eighth edition of *Olds' Maternal-Newborn Nursing & Women's Health Across the Lifespan.*

CARE DURING ADMISSION AND FIRST 4 HOURS OF LIFE

You enter the birthing room to meet Ryan and his parents. Ryan is 20 minutes old and is in a quiet, alert state while interacting with his mother.

1. What seven essential areas of information would you ascertain about Ryan's perinatal, intranatal, and immediate postnatal period to be placed on the newborn's chart?

   a.

   b.

   c.

   d.

   e.

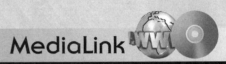

MediaLink

http://www.prenhall.com/davidson

Additional resources for this content can be found on the Student DVD-ROM accompanying the eighth edition of *Olds' Maternal-Newborn Nursing & Women's Health Across the Lifespan,* and on the Companion Website at http://www.prenhall.com/davidson. Click on the text chapter number(s) listed for this content to select the appropriate activities.

Prentice Hall Nursing MediaLink DVD-ROM
- Audio Glossary
- NCLEX Review
- Nursing in Action: Breastfeeding
- Nursing in Action: Thermoregulation of the Newborn
- Video: Newborn Care
- Tools: Actions and Effects of Selected Drugs Used During Breastfeeding

Companion Website
- Additional NCLEX Review
- Case Study: Newborn Care
- Case Study: Breastfeeding Client
- Care Plan Activity: Infant Care During Transition
- Care Plan Activity: Initial Newborn Care
- Care Plan Activity: Breastfeeding Concerns
- Tools: Actions and Effects of Selected Drugs Used During Breastfeeding

     f.

     g.

2. List and prioritize eight nursing actions you would carry out during the admission process and first 4 hours (transitional period) of the newborn's life.

     a.

     b.

     c.

     d.

     e.

     f.

     g.

     h.

3. Why is a vitamin K medication given prophylactically to newborns?

     The appropriate dose of Vitamin K is _____.

4. **Critical Thinking in Practice:** The following action sequence is designed to help you think through basic clinical problems.

   Prakash, a 3450-g baby boy, is born breech to Mrs. Balasubraniyam and has an Apgar score of 7 at 1 minute. Mrs. Balasubraniyam has requested to begin the bonding process by breastfeeding Prakash on the birthing bed.

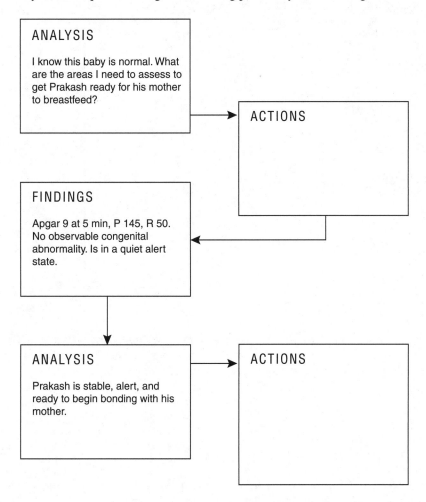

5. A nurse is administering vitamin K (AquaMEPHYTON) to a newborn. Which site is most appropriate for the injection?

   a. Deltoid

   b. Dorsogluteal

   c. Vastus lateralis

   d. Ventrogluteal

6. Prophylactic eye ointments are instilled in the newborn's eyes in the immediate newborn period to prevent

   (a) _____, which is caused by (b) _____.

7. List two prophylactic eye ointments that are commonly used.

   a.

   b.

At the end of the transitional period, or 4 to 6 hours after birth, baseline laboratory tests are completed.

8. For each of the following laboratory values, identify the significance and appropriate nursing interventions:

Laboratory Value	Significance	Nursing Interventions
Central hematocrit of 68%		
Hemoglobin of 12.5 g/dL		
Bilirubin of 15 mg/dL		
Heel-stick glucose less than 45 mg%		

9. While working in the nursery, you notice that baby Andrew, age 5 hours, has turned blue. Closer inspection reveals a large amount of frothy mucus in his mouth. What would be your nursing diagnosis in this situation? What immediate nursing interventions would you undertake?

Ryan Montoya has successfully progressed through the transitional period; he is now 6 hours old and continues to be adapting well to extrauterine life.

NEWBORN NURSING ASSESSMENTS FOLLOWING TRANSITION

10. You are assigned to the mother-baby area. List six daily assessments that are made of each newborn.

a.

b.

c.

d.

e.

f.

11. Ryan is now 12 hours old. He voids as you begin to change his diaper. What observations should you make about his voiding?

12. If Ryan had failed to void within 24 hours after birth, describe the assessments you would carry out.

13. Within how many hours after birth would you expect Ryan to have his first stool and what would its appearance initially be?

BREASTFEEDING

14. Helena Montoya wants to breastfeed Ryan. She tells you that she is really interested in breastfeeding but feels overwhelmed because she has so many questions and feels uncertain about beginning. She states, "I feel so full of questions that I wonder if I will ever know what to do." Based on your analysis of this data, formulate a nursing diagnosis that might apply. (See Chapter 31.)

15. Based on your diagnosis, what information would you give Helena about breastfeeding her son?

    a. Methods for encouraging the baby to breastfeed

    b. Latching on

    c. Breaking suction before removing the infant from the breast

    d. Frequency of feeding

16. The nurse assesses the mother holding the infant tucked under her arm with the infant's back and shoulders in her palm. How would the nurse document this feeding position?

    a. Cradling

    b. Football

    c. Lap

    d. Side-lying

17. A new breastfeeding mother is concerned about her small breasts, and whether she can produce enough milk. The nurse teaches the mother that the best indication that her baby is receiving adequate nutrition is that the baby

    a. is hungry and wants to eat every 2–3 hours.

    b. sleeps for 4–6 hours between feedings.

    c. gains 2 ounces per week.

    d. has 6–8 wet diapers.

18. You stay and assist Helena with breastfeeding and answer her questions. Once she appears comfortable, you leave, but you check back with her periodically. Later in the morning when her baby is sleeping, you return to share information about other areas related to successful breastfeeding. What information would you share with Helena about the following areas?

    a. Expression and storing of breast milk

    b. Environmental influences on successful breastfeeding

    c. Use of medications while breastfeeding

    d. External support systems

19. Helena is scheduled to remain on postpartum for only 24 to 48 hours. What actions can you take to help reinforce her learning so that things will go more smoothly when she is home?

20. How will you evaluate the effectiveness of your teaching plan in meeting Helena's education needs?

21. A Korean client has just delivered and has stated that she would like to breastfeed. What is the nurse's best response to the client's comment, "I do not want to breastfeed until my milk supply is well established"?

    a. "Colostrum can build your newborn's immune system considerably. Would you like to reconsider?"

    b. "Here is some information about breastfeeding and current research that discusses the benefits. Please take some time to read this, and I will be back to discuss this with you."

    c. "I think it is best to ensure a strong milk supply immediately. Putting your newborn to breast right now will assist with that."

    d. "What are your thoughts and preferences about breastfeeding? I would like to help you with this process in any way that I can."

Christy is a 2-day-old, formula-fed, 3175-g infant. During a follow-up call, her mother is concerned because "she takes only 1 1/2 oz at each feeding."

22. What would your response be?

23. A nursery nurse is teaching the parents of an 8-pound, 4-ounce baby about appropriate nutritional intake. How many ounces of formula should this baby have each day?

    a. 5–18 ounces per day

    b. 19–22 ounces per day

    c. 24–28 ounces per day

    d. 29–33 ounces per day

24. Which behavior observed by the nurse indicates good bottle-feeding technique? The mother (Select all that apply.)

    a. enlarges the nipple hole to allow for a steady stream of formula to flow.

    b. keeps the infant close with the head elevated.

    c. keeps the nipple full of formula throughout the feeding.

    d. points the bottle at the infant's tongue.

    e. props the bottle on a rolled towel.

25. On your mother-baby unit, you are conducting mothers' classes on newborn characteristics. The mothers express concerns about the following common occurrences. How would you respond to each?

    a. "Can I hurt him by washing his hair over that soft spot? When will it close?"

    b. "All my family's eyes are brown, but her eyes are blue."

    c. "Why are there tiny white spots across the bridge of her nose and on her chin?"

d. "Are my baby's eyes all right? There are bright red marks on the white part of his eyes."

e. "He has white patches in his mouth. Is that milk? How can you determine the cause?"

f. "My son's breasts are so swollen. Will the swelling go down?"

g. "When I changed her diaper, there was blood on it."

h. "Are her feet clubbed? They turn in."

i. "Why does his head look funny? The bones of his head cross over each other and look so narrow on the sides."

j. List other questions you have been asked by mothers and your responses to them.

CIRCUMCISION

26. Before discharge, Ryan Montoya is circumcised using a plastibell. What are your nursing responsibilities before, during, and following the circumcision?

27. Nursing interventions for Ryan following his circumcision include

    a. administering an analgesic.

    b. applying a topical anesthetic to the site.

    c. keeping him in the nursery for 1 hour.

    d. loosely wrapping the diaper around him.

28. Michael, an uncircumcised newborn, is ready for discharge. What instructions should you give his parents about penile care?

29. In order to prevent infant abduction, what should be done with every parent-infant interaction?

    a. Having a parent come to the nursery to specifically point out her infant

    b. Matching the mother's room number to the bed card

    c. Visually matching identification bands

    d. Parental verbalization that this is their infant

DISCHARGE TEACHING/PREPARATION FOR CARE AT HOME

30. Nursing actions that help a new mother relate to her baby after birth include

    a. calling the infant by name as soon as possible after birth.

    b. feeding the infant the first few times so that the mother can see the procedure.

    c. strongly encouraging the mother to breastfeed.

    d. undressing the baby completely so that all body parts can be seen.

31. Which of the following behaviors by a new father would indicate "engrossment"?

    a. Being able to express disappointment about the sex of the child

    b. Being afraid of hurting the infant while holding the infant

    c. Noting the individual characteristics of the infant including molding

    d. Stating that he feels more mature after seeing his infant for the first time

32. You are to present a newborn discharge teaching program. List the essential components of this teaching program.

33. The nurse is evaluating discharge teaching. Which statement by the parents demonstrates an understanding of temperature assessment for an infant?

    a. "Her temperature needs to be taken only when she shows signs of illness."

    b. "She only needs to have her temperature taken when she feels warm to the touch."

    c. "We need to take her axillary temperature every day at home."

    d. "We should only take her rectal temperature at home if she is sick enough to go to the doctor."

34. Before discharge, what screening and immunizations procedures may be instituted?

35. For the trip home from the birthing center, the newborn would be adequately protected if transported in

    a. an appropriate car seat facing the rear seat of the car.

    b. an approved car seat facing forward in the middle of the rear seat.

    c. an infant carrier secured to the rear seat with a seat belt.

    d. the mother's arms while she is seated in the rear of the car.

36. Briefly identify some culturally based newborn care practices that you have encountered or you have seen in your family.

37. **Memory Check**: Define the following abbreviations.

    a. AC

    b. BAT

    c. CC

    d. HC

    e. PKU

CHAPTER 16

NURSING CARE OF NEWBORNS WITH CONDITIONS PRESENT AT BIRTH

The majority of pregnancies end with the birth of healthy term infants. However, some infants are at risk even before birth because of an altered intrauterine environment. Early nursing intervention can significantly improve the baby's outlook.

This chapter considers the factors that contribute to the development of an at-risk infant, the commonly used methods of assessing an infant's status, and, finally, the problems at-risk infants face.

This chapter corresponds to Chapter 32 in the eighth edition of *Olds' Maternal-Newborn Nursing & Women's Health Across the Lifespan.*

CLASSIFICATION OF AT-RISK INFANTS

1. Identify six maternal factors that may contribute to the birth of an at-risk infant.

   a.

   b.

   c.

   d.

   e.

   f.

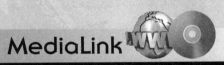

MediaLink

http://www.prenhall.com/
davidson

Additional resources for this content can be found on the Student DVD-ROM accompanying the eighth edition of *Olds' Maternal-Newborn Nursing & Women's Health Across the Lifespan,* and on the Companion Web Site at http://www.prenhall.com/davidson. Click on the text chapter number(s) listed for this content to select the appropriate activities.

Prentice Hall Nursing MediaLink DVD-ROM
- Audio Glossary
- NCLEX Review

Companion Web Site
- Additional NCLEX Review
- Case Study: Postterm Newborn
- Care Plan Activity: Infant of a Diabetic Mother

Using a neonatal classification and mortality chart, plot each newborn's gestational age and weight, and identify the appropriate classification for each of the following newborns (each newborn may belong to a classification group based on both gestational age and weight):

2. Baby Joey is at 36 to 37 weeks' gestation, twin B, weighing 1500 g.

   Classification _____

3. Baby Gwynn is at 42 1/2 weeks' gestation by clinical determination and weighs 3150 g.

   Classification _____

4. Baby Sara is 34 weeks and weighs 2060 g.

   Classification _____

5. Baby Fernando is a 39-week newborn weighing 3950 g.

   Classification _____

6. Baby Carla is 41 weeks and weighs 2500 g.

   Classification _____

7. In assessing the newborn for at-risk status, the nurse should know that

   a. any infant with a birth weight of less than 2500 g is preterm.

   b. gestational age is the one criterion utilized to establish mortality risk.

   c. infants who are preterm and small for gestational age have the highest mortality risk.

   d. the large-for-gestational-age infant has little risk of neonatal morbidity.

SMALL-FOR-GESTATIONAL-AGE (SGA) INFANT

8. List four conditions that can result in an SGA infant.

   a.

   b.

   c.

   d.

9. A newborn who is classified as small for gestational age must

   a. be at or below the 10th percentile on a gestational age/birth weight chart.

   b. be born before the 34th week of gestation.

   c. have suffered growth restriction secondary to placental malfunction.

   d. weigh less than 2500 g (5.5 lb).

10. A nurse is caring for a small-for-gestational age (SGA) newborn. For what complication is this baby at risk? (Select all that apply.)

    a. Hyperglycemia

    b. Hypoglycemia

    c. Polycythemia

    d. Aspiration syndrome

INFANT OF A DIABETIC MOTHER (IDM)

11. Richard is a 36-weeks-gestation newborn, weighing 9 lb, 1 oz. His admitting nursery information indicates that his mother is a gestational onset diabetic. What physical characteristics would you expect him to have?

12. Identify the cause for Richard's large size.

13. What laboratory test should be carried out on Richard and when?

14. Hypoglycemia occurs when blood glucose levels fall below _____ mg/dL.

15. A nurse is admitting an infant of a diabetic mother (IDM). At 1 hour of age, the nurse notices that the newborn is very jittery and has irregular respirations. Which action by the nurse is most appropriate?

    a. Begin oxygen by nasal cannula.

    b. Assess the newborn's blood glucose.

    c. Initiate use of a cardiac/apnea monitor.

    d. Place the newborn under a radiant warmer.

16. Identify the nursing interventions you would carry out relative to the assessment and treatment of hypoglycemia. (See text, Chapter 33.)

17. Richard is a newborn who experienced symptomatic hypoglycemia and required an IV infusion of dextrose. His condition has stabilized, and the physician has changed him to oral feedings. As Richard begins oral feedings, the nurse should anticipate that medical orders will include

   a. administering long-acting epinephrine.

   b. discontinuing IV after first formula feeding.

   c. giving a bolus infusion of 10% dextrose.

   d. reinstituting frequent glucose monitoring during transition.

18. The newborn infant of a class B (White's scale) diabetic mother is 25 minutes old. In comparison to infants of class D–F diabetic mothers (who have poor uterine blood supply), this baby is at higher risk for developing

   a. hypocalcemia.

   b. hyperbilirubinemia.

   c. polycythemia.

   d. respiratory distress.

POSTTERM INFANT

Answer as either true (T) or false (F).

19. _____ Postmature infants have special skin needs because of limited glycogen stores.

20. _____ Yellowish green nail beds result from meconium staining.

21. _____ Postmature infants are at risk for hyperglycemia.

22. _____ Meconium staining of the skin and intrauterine growth restriction are manifestations of postmaturity syndrome.

23. Like the preterm infant, the newborn with postmaturity syndrome is at high risk for cold stress due to

   a. absence of vernix.

   b. decreased subcutaneous fat.

   c. extended posture.

   d. parchment-like skin.

PRETERM INFANT

24. List four major causes of prematurity.

   a.

   b.

   c.

   d.

25. Which of the following characteristics is indicative of a preterm newborn of 34 weeks' gestation?

    a. The scalp hair is silky and lies in silky strands.

    b. The skin, except for the face, is covered with lanugo.

    c. The sole creases cover the anterior two thirds of the foot.

    d. The upper two thirds of the pinna curves inward.

26. A preterm infant arrives in the nursery. What three initial assessments should you make?

    a.

    b.

    c.

27. When auscultating the chest of a preterm newborn, the nurse hears crackles and a continuous systolic murmur with clicks at the base of the heart. The nurse should suspect the presence of

    a. bronchopulmonary dysplasia.

    b. patent ductus arteriosus.

    c. pulmonary atelectasis.

    d. ventricular septal defect.

28. If an infant experiences an apneic episode, the first nursing activity should be to

    a. apply gentle tactile stimulation.

    b. call the physician.

    c. increase the rate of prescribed oxygen.

    d. suction the mouth and nose with a bulb syringe.

29. The most common complication associated with preterm births is the development of

    a. bronchopulmonary dysplasia.

    b. periodic apnea.

    c. persistent fetal circulation.

    d. respiratory distress syndrome.

30. Briefly describe the benefits of each: early breast milk feedings (also see text, Chapter 31), minimal enteral nutrition, and premature formulas.

31. The parents of a 28-week-gestation newborn ask the nurse, "Why does he have to be fed through a tube in his mouth?" The nurse's best response is that

    a. "It allows us to accurately determine the baby's intake."

    b. "The baby's sucking, swallowing, and breathing are not coordinated yet."

    c. "The baby's stomach cannot digest formula at this time."

    d. "It helps to prevent thrush, an infection that could affect the baby's mouth."

Mary, a 34-week preterm infant, is initially maintained on IV fluids via umbilical catheter. When her respiratory status improves, she is placed on a half-strength premature formula via gavage feedings every 2 hours.

32. How would you assess proper placement of a gavage tube before feedings?

33. What nursing assessments would you make to determine Mary's tolerance of gavage feedings?

34. When Mary is 2 days old, her weight is average for gestational age (AGA). She is being carefully monitored before initiation of nipple feeding. Which of the following data groups would indicate that she is *not* ready for nipple feeding?

    a. Alert; axillary temperature of 97F

    b. Apical heart rate 120; skin temperature 36.5C

    c. Gaining weight; coordinated suck-swallow reflex

    d. Nasal flaring; sustained respiratory rate of 68

35. Briefly describe developmentally supportive nursing measures.

INFANT OF SUBSTANCE-ABUSING MOTHER

36. What common complications may be associated with cocaine-exposed infants?

37. Claire, a 2-day-old, 3100-g newborn, is observed to be going through withdrawal. Her 18-year-old mother was addicted to heroin during the pregnancy. List six symptoms of withdrawal you may observe in Claire.

    a.

    b.

    c.

    d.

    e.

    f.

38. The nursing management of a heroin-addicted newborn experiencing withdrawal includes

    a. administration of methadone and frequent assessment of vital signs.

    b. frequent assessment of vital signs and wrapping the infant snugly in a blanket.

    c. meticulous skin and perineal care and frequent tactile stimulation.

    d. minimal tactile stimulation and the provision of loose, nonrestrictive clothing.

39. During the past week, Claire has been irritable and eating poorly. She has not gained weight since birth. The physician orders phenobarbital for her. How many milligrams will the nurse administer per dose?

    a. 6 mg

    b. 12 mg

    c. 24 mg

    d. 36 mg

40. The nurse is teaching a preconception class. One class participant asks the nurse if one glass of wine at dinner each night is all right. The most appropriate nursing response is

    a. "The first 3 months of pregnancy are the most critical for fetal development, and alcohol should be avoided during that period."

    b. "There has been no minimal amount of alcohol determined to be safe in pregnancy."

    c. "This is a minimal amount and should not harm your baby."

    d. "To avoid alcohol withdrawal in your baby, refrain from any alcohol during the last 3 months."

41. What are the special needs of the drug-exposed infant at home?

REFLECTIONS

Think about an at-risk newborn you have taken care of. What were the parents' responses? Describe what the experience was like for you.

_____

_____

_____

_____

_____

_____

_____

NEWBORN AT RISK FOR HIV/AIDS

42. Nursing interventions for an infant at risk for AIDS include

    a. a quiet, dim environment.

    b. feeding with 24 cal/oz formula.

    c. frequent, gentle handling.

    d. tight swaddling.

43. What instructions for care in the home should be given to parents of an infant at risk for AIDS?

44. When teaching home care to parents of an HIV-infected baby, the mother says, "My baby had diarrhea when I was holding him in my bed with me. What should I do with my sheets?" The nurse should tell her to

    a. place them in two plastic bags, tie them securely, and put them in the trash.

    b. wash them in hot, sudsy water, separate from other household laundry.

    c. wash them in hot, sudsy water along with other household laundry.

    d. wash them separately in hot, sudsy water containing household bleach.

45. **Memory Check:** Define the following abbreviations.

   a. AIDS

   b. ARBD

   c. FAS

   d. IDM

   e. ISAM

   f. IUGR

   g. LGA

   h. SGA

CHAPTER 17

NURSING CARE OF NEWBORNS WITH BIRTH-RELATED STRESSORS

This chapter focuses on many of the problems that may afflict high-risk infants, with emphasis on nursing assessment and interventions and, finally, on evaluation of effectiveness of care.

Some infants develop serious problems during their early hours and days of life. The maternal or fetal factors that increase the baby's risk can be predicted during the antepartal period. In other cases, the infant's risk status results from insults or complications that occur during labor and birth.

This chapter corresponds to Chapter 33 in the eighth edition of *Olds' Maternal-Newborn Nursing & Women's Health Across the Lifespan.*

RESUSCITATION

In addition to providing warmth, immediate newborn care for all at-risk newborns is centered around determining the need for resuscitation.

1. Dava Walker has a previous obstetric history of fetal death of undetermined cause at 8 months' gestation. After the physician obtains a fetal scalp blood pH of 7.22, baby boy Walker is born. Which action by the nurse is the appropriate *initial* newborn resuscitation step?

    a. Inflating the lungs with positive pressure

    b. Inserting a nasogastric tube

    c. Positioning the head in the "sniffing position"

    d. Suctioning the oropharynx and nasopharynx

2. Baby Ken, a 43 1/2-week postterm newborn, experienced early deceleration in labor. Yellow-green amniotic fluid was present at the time of membrane rupture.

    a. Ken is at risk for what neonatal problem?

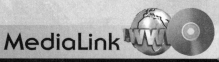

MediaLink

http://www.prenhall.com/davidson

Additional resources for this content can be found on the Student DVD-ROM accompanying the eighth edition of *Olds' Maternal-Newborn Nursing & Women's Health Across the Lifespan,* and on the Companion Website at http://www.prenhall.com/davidson. Click on the text chapter number(s) listed for this content to select the appropriate activities.

Prentice Hall Nursing MediaLink DVD-ROM

*   Audio Glossary
*   NCLEX Review

Companion Website

*   Additional NCLEX Review
*   Case Study: Newborn with Jaundice
*   Care Plan Activity: Infection in a Newborn

b. What resuscitative measures should be instituted as soon as his head and face appear on the perineum?

c. What additional resuscitative measures or actions do you anticipate will be carried out after Ken is born?

3. **Critical Thinking Challenge:** The following situation has been included to challenge your critical thinking. Read the situation, then answer the question "yes" or "no," and give the rationale for your decision.

Celeste, a 3200-g term baby, is born vaginally. The amniotic fluid is lightly meconium stained. She was suctioned on the perineum and cried vigorously within 30 seconds of birth.

Is Celeste a candidate for further resuscitation measures?

Yes _____   No _____

Explain your answer:

Brian, a term baby, was born vaginally 2 hours after his mother received 75 mg of meperidine (Demerol) IM. He has some flexion of extremities and acrocyanosis, HR-96, slow and irregular respiratory effort, and facial grimace. His Apgar score at 1 min is 5. You are assisting the physician/neonatal nurse practitioner with the resuscitation.

4. Why is deep, vigorous suctioning of the airways to be avoided?

5. During bag-and-mask resuscitation you watch Brian's resuscitation bag to ensure it is inflating adequately, and you watch the pressure manometer to achieve the desired pressure of (a) _____ cm H_2O at a rate of (b)_____ times per minute.

6. Based on Brian's intrapartal history, what other resuscitative measures does he need?

7. The *first* pharmacologic agent given in the chemical resuscitation phase of neonatal resuscitation is

   a. a volume expander, to maintain blood pressure.

   b. dopamine, to correct metabolic acidosis.

   c. epinephrine, to stimulate the heart.

   d. sodium bicarbonate, to correct respiratory acidosis.

On April 18 at 1:45 PM, a 35-week, 1580-g male infant named Julio was born to a 20-year-old primigravida.

8. Julio is beginning to show signs of respiratory distress. Determine the priority for the following nursing interventions:

   1. Notify the physician.

   2. If cyanosis occurs, provide oxygen.

   3. Record time, symptoms, degree of symptoms, and whether oxygen relieved the symptoms of respiratory distress.

   4. Apply monitoring electrodes.

   5. Maintain a patent airway.

      a. 2, 1, 5, 4, and 3

      b. 5, 1, 2, 3, and 4

      c. 4, 2, 5, 1, and 3

      d. 5, 2, 1, 4, and 3

RESPIRATORY DISTRESS SYNDROME

Tricia, a 3 1/2-lb (1587-g) newborn with a gestational age of 34 weeks, was born at 10:30 PM. Her Apgar score at 1 minute was 3, necessitating resuscitation via intubation and oxygen administration. On admission to the NICU, her vital signs are pulse 150, respirations 50, and rectal temperature of 96.2F (35.7C). She is placed in a radiant heat warmer, and an umbilical artery catheter is inserted for IV infusion.

9. Tricia develops respiratory distress syndrome (RDS) 3 hours after birth. What would be an assessment finding? (Select all that apply.)

   a. Feeding intolerance

   b. Increased blood pressure

   c. Nasal flaring

   d. Retractions

10. Additional physical assessment data on Tricia's respiratory status reveal minimal nasal flaring, chest lag on inspiration with just visible intercostal (lower chest) and xiphoid retractions, and audible expiratory grunting. Using the Silverman-Andersen index (Figure 17–1), your respiratory distress score for Tricia would be _____.

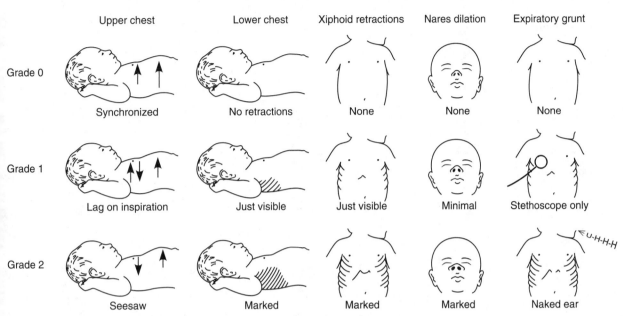

Figure 17–1   Evaluation of respiratory status using the Silverman-Andersen index.
SOURCE: From Ross Laboratories, Nursing Inservice Aid no. 2, Columbus, Ohio; and Silverman, W. A., & Andersen, D. H. (1956). Pediatrics, 17, 1. Copyright © 1956: American Academy of Pediatrics.

11. What three factors may predispose Tricia to develop respiratory distress syndrome?

    a.

    b.

    c.

12. Tricia's respirations are now 65 per minute; she has an apical pulse of 152 to 176 beats per minute; and her arterial blood gases show a pH of 7.3, PO_2 of 55 mmHg, and PCO_2 of 69 mmHg. What are your nursing responsibilities during oxygen administration and how can you evaluate the effectiveness of the oxygen therapy?

13. As Tricia's respiratory distress decreases, monitoring her respiratory status can be accomplished by noninvasive methods. Complete the following chart on noninvasive oxygen monitoring techniques.

Technique	Desired Range	Action	Nursing Responsibilities
Transcutaneous oxygen monitor (TCM)			
Pulse oximetry			

14. Tricia's oxygen concentration is carefully regulated, based on her PO_2 and PCO_2 levels, because high blood levels of oxygen

   a. cause cardiac shunt closures, although the latter are not permanent.

   b. cause peripheral circulatory collapse.

   c. may cause retinal spasms, leading to the development of retinopathy of prematurity.

   d. may produce hyperbilirubinemia.

COLD STRESS

At-risk infants are susceptible to temperature instability and should be placed in a regulated neutral thermal environment. If the infant's thermal environment is not maintained, cold stress can occur.

15. What four metabolic changes and resultant problems may occur as a result of cold stress?

   a.

   b.

   c.

   d.

16. Which of the following blood gases might be found in a newborn with extreme cold stress after birth?

    a. pH 7.35, PCO_2 36, PO_2 98, HCO_3 26

    b. pH 7.37, PCO_2 32, PO_2 98, HCO_3 26

    c. pH 7.19, PCO_2 44, PO_2 50, HCO_3 18

    d. pH 7.19, PCO_2 58, PO_2 60, HCO_3 24

17. A newborn has experienced cold stress. Which of the following nursing actions should be included in the baby's care plan?

    a. Initiate Dextrostix monitoring of blood glucose levels.

    b. Monitor rectal temperature hourly.

    c. Rapidly infuse 50% dextrose IV per standing protocol (or obtain order for).

    d. Using radiant warmer, institute measures for rapid temperature elevation.

NEONATAL JAUNDICE

18. Identify the characteristics of pathologic jaundice as related to causes, time of onset, and bilirubin level in the term newborn.

19. An African American mother asks how to assess for jaundice in her newborn. Which of the following is the most appropriate answer for the nurse to offer?

    a. "A good place to look is the inside of the mouth. Use a good light to help you see."

    b. "Pressing the sole of your baby's foot is helpful. If it blanches yellow, then the baby is considered jaundiced."

    c. "Such an assessment is best done by the doctor. She knows how to identify jaundice."

    d. "The best way to assess your baby is to check the white part of the eyes. If jaundice is present, they will have a yellow color."

20. What factors might influence your assessment of the newborn's developing jaundice?

21. Sally Hines is a primipara whose baby has developed jaundice as a result of ABO incompatibility. Because it is her first pregnancy, Sally cannot understand why her baby is affected. The nurse's best response would be based on which of the following statements?

    a. Anti-A and anti-B antibodies are naturally occurring; thus, they can affect a first pregnancy.

    b. Because she has had no previous pregnancies, Sally must have had a blood transfusion with incompatible blood.

    c. It is rare for the newborn with a first pregnancy to experience hemolytic disease.

    d. With ABO incompatibility, the mother becomes sensitized early in pregnancy; thus a first pregnancy can be affected.

22. **Critical Thinking in Practice:** The following action sequence is designed to help you think through a clinical problem pertaining to hemolytic disease of the newborn.

    You are taking care of Alice, a 24-hour-old, 7 lb, 2 oz newborn, and her mother on the mother-baby unit. During your initial assessments and care of Alice, you notice she looks yellow.

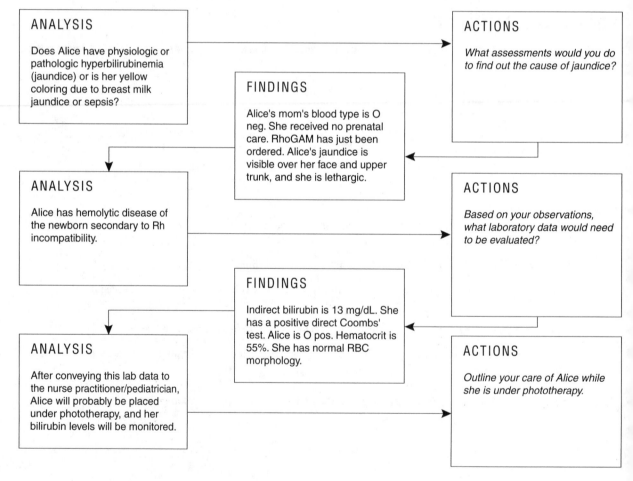

ANALYSIS

Does Alice have physiologic or pathologic hyperbilirubinemia (jaundice) or is her yellow coloring due to breast milk jaundice or sepsis?

ACTIONS

What assessments would you do to find out the cause of jaundice?

FINDINGS

Alice's mom's blood type is O neg. She received no prenatal care. RhoGAM has just been ordered. Alice's jaundice is visible over her face and upper trunk, and she is lethargic.

ANALYSIS

Alice has hemolytic disease of the newborn secondary to Rh incompatibility.

ACTIONS

Based on your observations, what laboratory data would need to be evaluated?

FINDINGS

Indirect bilirubin is 13 mg/dL. She has a positive direct Coombs' test. Alice is O pos. Hematocrit is 55%. She has normal RBC morphology.

ANALYSIS

After conveying this lab data to the nurse practitioner/pediatrician, Alice will probably be placed under phototherapy, and her bilirubin levels will be monitored.

ACTIONS

Outline your care of Alice while she is under phototherapy.

23. A newborn undergoing phototherapy experiences increased urine output and loose stools. The nurse should

    a. decrease the phototherapy unit's level of irradiance.

    b. immediately discontinue phototherapy.

    c. provide extra fluids to prevent dehydration.

    d. recognize this is a normal occurrence needing no intervention.

24. While receiving phototherapy lights, babies should

    a. be unclothed with the eyes shielded.

    b. be unclothed with the eyes and genitals shielded.

    c. not be removed from under the lights until treatment is completed.

    d. not be disturbed by frequent parental visits.

NEWBORN WITH ANEMIA OR POLYCYTHEMIA

25. A nursing care plan for an anemic newborn should most likely include

    a. administering oxygen.

    b. giving IV push calcium gluconate.

    c. managing phototherapy treatments.

    d. monitoring cardiac and respiratory function.

26. For a newborn with polycythemia, which of the following laboratory results would indicate that medical therapy is effective?

    a. Central venous hematocrit of 70%

    b. Central venous hematocrit of 55%

    c. Serum calcium level of 8 mg/dL

    d. Venous hemoglobin of 25 g/dL

27. A nurse is preparing to perform a heel stick for a capillary hematocrit. How can the nurse decrease the chance of obtaining a falsely high value?

    a. Be careful not to shake the capillary tube after filling it.

    b. Do not perform the heel stick during or soon after a crying episode.

    c. Obtain the blood within 30 minutes after a feeding.

    d. Warm the heel before obtaining the blood.

NEONATAL INFECTIONS

28. You are taking care of Haruko, who is 2 days old, and you note that he is increasingly lethargic and refuses to eat. He is diagnosed as having sepsis neonatorum. List four factors that increase the newborn's susceptibility to infections.

    a.

    b.

    c.

    d.

29. Identify two bacterial organisms that may cause sepsis neonatorum.

    a.

    b.

30. On admission to the nursery, it is noted that the mother's membranes were ruptured for 48 hours before delivery and her temperature is 102F (38.9C). What information from this newborn's assessment should the nurse evaluate further?

    a. Axillary temperature 97.2F (36.2C)

    b. Excessive bruising of presenting part

    c. Irregular respiratory rate

    d. Jitteriness

31. What are your nursing responsibilities while caring for a septic newborn? Include your rationale.

32. The most common congenitally acquired viral infection is

    a. cytomegalovirus.

    b. herpes simplex virus.

    c. syphilis.

33. What would you do to facilitate attachment between parents and their at-risk infant?

34. What discharge instruction and arrangements should be made before Mary's parents take her home?

35. **Memory Check:** Define the following abbreviations:

   a. BPD

   b. MAS

   c. NTE

   d. RDS

   e. UAC

CHAPTER 18

NURSING ASSESSMENT AND CARE OF THE POSTPARTAL FAMILY

The postpartal period is a time of major physiologic and psychologic adaptations as the body completes its adjustment following childbirth. This chapter begins with questions on common physiologic and psychologic changes and moves to clinical application of the nursing process in providing care for the postpartal family.

This chapter corresponds to Chapters 34 and 35 in the eighth edition of *Olds' Maternal-Newborn Nursing & Women's Health Across the Lifespan.*

POSTPARTUM CHANGES

1. Discuss physiologic and psychologic changes that occur in the postpartal period (puerperium).

ATTACHMENT IMMEDIATELY AFTER BIRTH

2. Denise and Dan just had their first baby 10 minutes ago. What stage of labor and birth are they in?

3. Denise and Dan are exhibiting beginning attachment behaviors. What will you observe?

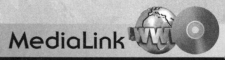

MediaLink

http://www.prenhall.com/davidson

Additional resources for this content can be found on the Student DVD-ROM accompanying the eighth edition of *Olds' Maternal-Newborn Nursing & Women's Health Across the Lifespan,* and on the Companion Website at http://www.prenhall.com/davidson. Click on the text chapter number(s) listed for this content to select the appropriate activities.

Prentice Hall Nursing MediaLink DVD-ROM
- Audio Glossary
- NCLEX Review

Companion Website
- Additional NCLEX Review
- Case Study: Mother-Infant Bonding
- Case Study: Postpartum Client
- Care Plan Activity: Postpartal Care Following Vaginal Birth
- Care Plan Activity: Postpartal Care Following Cesarean Birth

4. How can you support the attachment process at this time?

PHYSIOLOGIC POSTPARTAL CHANGES

5. The fundus should be

   a. at the level of the symphysis pubis.

   b. at the level of the umbilicus.

   c. midway between the umbilicus and symphysis pubis.

   d. two fingerbreadths below the umbilicus.

6. The lochia should have a

   a. characteristic foul odor and consist of blood mixed with a small amount of mucus.

   b. characteristic foul odor and a dark brown color with occasional red bleeding.

   c. fleshy odor and be clear-colored and moderate in amount.

   d. fleshy odor with blood and a small amount of mucus mixed in.

7. The perineum should be

   a. edematous, painful to pressure, and displaying a clear discharge.

   b. edematous, painful to pressure, and perhaps displaying hemorrhoids.

   c. displaying clear drainage and perhaps hemorrhoids.

   d. intensely painful in the episiotomy area and displaying clear drainage.

8. The breasts should be

   a. engorged and not secreting any fluid.

   b. engorged and secreting colostrum.

   c. soft and secreting colostrum.

   d. soft and secreting milk.

9. Uterine involution occurs as a result of

   a. a decrease in the number of myometrial cells.

   b. autolysis of protein material within the uterine wall.

   c. necrosis of the hypertrophic myometrial cells.

   d. necrotic degeneration of the placental site.

10. Explain the physiologic mechanisms that cause each of the following:

    a. Postpartal chill

    b. Postpartal diaphoresis

    c. Afterpains

11. During the postpartal period, what psychologic adaptations does a new mother face?

12. Describe *postpartum blues.*

MATERNAL ROLE ATTAINMENT

13. Name and briefly describe the four stages of maternal role attainment.

    a.

    b.

    c.

    d.

ASSESSMENT OF THE POSTPARTAL WOMAN

14. Identify nine areas that should be examined during the initial postpartal *physical* assessment and then at least daily until the woman is discharged. (Do not include psychologic assessment or information needs.)

    a.

    b.

    c.

    d.

    e.

    f.

    g.

    h.

    i.

15. Describe three observations you should make in assessing the breasts of a woman postpartally. Include your rationale for each.

    a.

    b.

    c.

16. The fundus is assessed following childbirth.

    a. Why is it necessary?

    b. Why is the client asked to empty her bladder before you assess her fundus?

    c. Describe the correct procedure for evaluating descent of the fundus.

    d. How is fundal height recorded (according to your agency's policy)?

17. Soon Yee, a 21-year-old primipara, gave birth 4 hours ago. Immediately following birth her fundus was midway between the symphysis and the umbilicus. Where would you expect it to be now?

18. What characteristics should you note in assessing Soon's lochia?

19. How do you record your findings about her lochia (according to your agency's policy)?

20. Soon reports that she got up to use the bathroom a short time ago and noticed a sudden increase in her lochia. From your check you know that her fundus is firm. How would you explain this occurrence to her?

21. In preparation for assessing Soon's perineum, you would have her assume the _____ position.

22. What observations about the condition of the client's anal area should be made during the assessment of the perineum?

23. What information regarding the client's urinary elimination should you elicit during your physical assessment?

24. What information about your client's intestinal elimination should you elicit during your physical assessment?

25. Discuss the teaching implications of your findings on intestinal elimination.

26. Why is it important to include an evaluation of your client's lower extremities as part of your postpartal assessment?

27. How is Homans' sign elicited?

28. **Critical Thinking in Practice:** The following action sequence is designed to help you think through basic clinical problems.

   Kay Sams gave birth at 0400. At 0830 you are completing her morning postpartum assessment. You find her fundus at one fingerbreadth above the umbilicus and displaced to the right side.

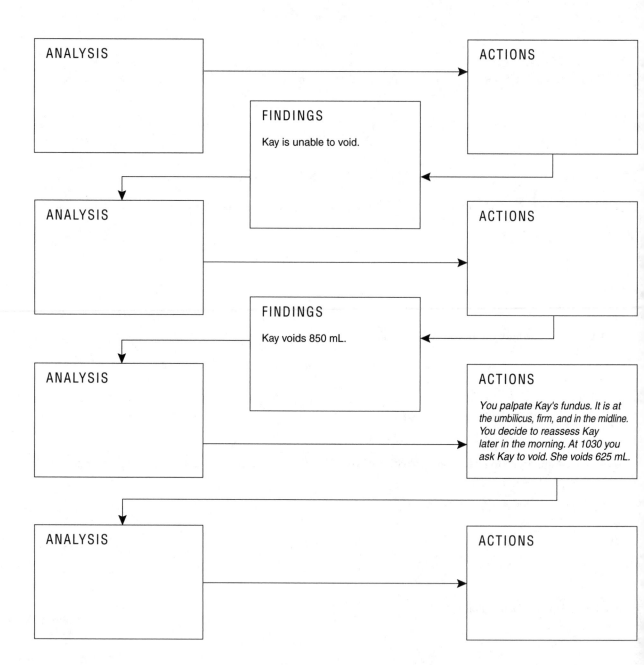

ANALYSIS

ACTIONS

FINDINGS

Kay is unable to void.

ANALYSIS

ACTIONS

FINDINGS

Kay voids 850 mL.

ANALYSIS

ACTIONS

You palpate Kay's fundus. It is at the umbilicus, firm, and in the midline. You decide to reassess Kay later in the morning. At 1030 you ask Kay to void. She voids 625 mL.

ANALYSIS

ACTIONS

29. What assessments are important in evaluating your client's nutritional status?

REFLECTIONS

Think about a woman you have cared for postpartally or someone you have visited soon after the birth of a child (perhaps this may apply to you). What were her emotions like? Did she share her feelings with you? Did she show any signs of the postpartum blues?

_____

_____

_____

_____

_____

_____

_____

30. Discuss factors you should consider in completing a psychologic assessment postpartally.

RELIEF OF POSTPARTAL DISCOMFORTS

31. For each of the discomforts in the following list, identify two comfort measures.

    a. Episiotomy/Laceration

    b. Hemorrhoids

    c. Afterpains

SUPPRESSION OF LACTATION

32. Suppression of lactation in nonbreastfeeding mothers is generally accomplished by mechanical methods. Explain these methods.

33. You are assisting Edna Lewis to the bathroom for the first time following childbirth.

    a. What nursing assessments should you make before Edna gets up?

    b. What teaching regarding perineal hygiene should you initiate at this time?

    c. Edna decides to remain in the bathroom and take a shower after she voids. What precautions should you take to ensure her safety?

PSYCHOLOGIC RESPONSES

34. Identify factors that influence a new mother's psychologic adjustment to childbirth and her newborn.

35. How can a nurse provide emotional support during this time?

36. You are caring for a woman who gave birth to a healthy infant 14 hours ago. When you enter her room, she is crying. She states, "I don't know what's wrong with me. I feel as let down as if it were the day after Christmas, and I can't seem to stop crying. What's going on? Do you know why I'm acting like this?" How would you respond?

37. Kate and Joe Clark express concern about the possible reaction of their 3-year-old son Tanner to the birth of their daughter. Briefly describe some actions they might take to help Tanner more easily adjust to the arrival of his sister.

38. In many postpartal units the focus of care and attention is the mother and her newborn. Describe how you would incorporate the father or support person into your focus of care.

39. In addition to her name, age, and social history, what information would you consider essential to have as part of your database in planning care for a woman postpartally?

40. Carla Roberts, age 29, gravida 3, para 2, gave birth to an 8 lb 7 oz boy at 4:15 AM. Her labor lasted 18 hours, and the baby was born by low forceps. She received no medication during labor but did have a pudendal block for birth. She had a midline episiotomy with a third-degree extension. She also has two large hemorrhoids. The baby had an Apgar score of 7 at 1 minute and 9 at 5 minutes. He is apparently healthy, although he has a large bruise on each temple from the forceps and pronounced molding of his head. The labor nurse reported that Harry Roberts, Carla's husband, was present at the birth and expressed great pleasure at the birth of his third son. Carla was openly disappointed that the newborn was not the girl she had so greatly desired.

It is now 8:00 AM. Carla has just finished breakfast, and you are assigned as her nurse today. Carla has voided twice since birth: 700 mL and 550 mL. Her fundus has remained firm and is at the umbilicus. Her lochia is rubra and moderate. Her vital signs are normal, and she is a breastfeeding mother. Her orders include a shower; a sitz bath tid; Dermoplast spray prn, up ad lib; Tylenol No. 3 every 4 hours prn; a regular diet; fluids; a straight catheter ×1 prn for marked distention; and Surfak 1 capsule bid. She is to be discharged at noon unless complications arise.

   a. What do you consider the highest priorities in planning Carla's physical care?

   b. What behaviors might Carla exhibit that would suggest possible failure to attach?

POSTPARTAL CARE OF THE WOMAN FOLLOWING CESAREAN BIRTH

41. How does postpartal assessment and care differ for the woman who gives birth by cesarean?

42. Patient-controlled analgesia (PCA) is becoming increasingly popular.

   a. Describe how it is used.

   b. How is the client on PCA protected from overdose?

CARE OF THE ADOLESCENT MOTHER

43. Describe some of the special nursing needs of the adolescent mother postpartally.

44. How can the postpartum nurse provide support and assistance to a woman who is relinquishing her infant?

DISCHARGE TEACHING

45. Lori and David Curtis are preparing to take their first child, Ella, home at 2:00 PM. Lori is planning to formula-feed Ella. Lori had an uncomplicated labor and birth but has a small midline episiotomy that has caused some discomfort. You are assigned to Mrs. Curtis today and are responsible for discharge teaching. Describe what information you will include in your discharge teaching for the following areas:

a. Care of the episiotomy

b. Rest

c. Activity and exercises

d. Resumption of sexual activity and birth control methods

e. Symptoms in the mother that should be reported

f. Support systems

g. Baby care

h. Symptoms in the baby that should be reported

i. Infant safety (crib, car seat)

j. Follow-up medical care for both mother and infant

k. Community resources

46. LaTisha Carson gave birth to her first child in the birthing room 6 hours ago. Now she is preparing for discharge. Describe how you will explain the reasons for and importance of returning to the hospital for a test for phenylketonuria and other metabolic disorders.

CHAPTER 19

HOME CARE OF THE POSTPARTAL FAMILY

Home care is an important component of childbearing nursing practice. The mother and newborn have been stabilized, and the parents have had opportunities to establish their beginning family in the birth center or hospital.

This chapter emphasizes continued assessment, anticipated findings and their significance, and appropriate nursing interventions. Questions related to evaluation are also included to provide guidelines for determining the effectiveness of care.

This chapter corresponds to Chapter 36 in the eighth edition of *Olds' Maternal-Newborn Nursing & Women's Health Across the Lifespan.*

HOME VISITS

1. The three areas of focus for a home visit to a postpartal family include

   a.

   b.

   c.

2. How is a postpartal home visit different from community health visits?

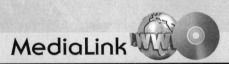

MediaLink

http://www.prenhall.com/davidson

Additional resources for this content can be found on the Student DVD-ROM accompanying the eighth edition of *Olds' Maternal-Newborn Nursing & Women's Health Across the Lifespan,* and on the Companion Website at http://www.prenhall.com/davidson. Click on the text chapter number(s) listed for this content to select the appropriate activities.

Prentice Hall Nursing MediaLink DVD-ROM
- Audio Glossary
- NCLEX Review
- Tools: Actions and Effects of Selected Drugs Used During Breastfeeding

Companion Website
- Additional NCLEX Review
- Case Study: Follow-up with the Client at Home
- Care Plan Activity: Breastfeeding Pain in a New Mother
- Tools: Actions and Effects of Selected Drugs Used During Breastfeeding

3. Identify five actions a nurse should take to ensure personal safety during a home visit.

   a.

   b.

   c.

   d.

   e.

4. What should the nurse do if he or she begins to feel unsafe during a home visit?

HOME CARE OF THE NEWBORN

5. Which of the following holding methods is recommended when shampooing the infant?

   a. Cradle hold

   b. Football hold

   c. Upright position

6. Why should the infant's resting position be changed periodically, especially during the early months of life?

7. Identify at least one reason for positioning a newborn infant on her or his back.

8. You are on a home visit to Elena Galez and her newborn daughter, Rose. Mrs. Galez asks when she can switch from sponge baths to tub baths. How would you respond?

9. What information should you give Mrs. Galez about assessment of Rose's umbilical cord?

10. The newborn's temperature should be taken by the _____ route.

For each of the following statements about newborn care, indicate **T** if the statement is true and **F** if it is false.

11. _____   Newborns should be given a daily bath.

12. _____   The eyes are washed from the inner to the outer canthus.

13. _____   The ear canal should be cleaned regularly with a cotton swab.

14. _____   Talcum powder is applied generously to help keep the infant's skin dry.

15. _____   The genital area should be cleansed daily with soap and water and with water after each wet or dirty diaper.

16. _____   The foreskin of uncircumcised infants should be gently retracted each day.

17. _____   If necessary, the newborn's nails may be trimmed straight across.

18. Complete the following chart comparing the stools of breastfed and formula-fed infants:

Characteristics of Stools	Breastfed	Formula-Fed
Frequency		
Color		
Consistency		
Odor		

HOME CARE OF THE POSTPARTAL WOMAN AND FAMILY

19. List four physical and developmental tasks the new mother must accomplish during the postpartal period.

    a.

    b.

    c.

    d.

20. Summarize areas of assessment the nurse should complete on the new mother during a postpartal home visit.

    a. Physical assessment

    b. Psychosocial assessment

For each of the following physical findings in the postpartal woman, indicate with a "**1**" those that are normally found at the first postpartal home visit and with a "**6**" those that are normally found by 6 weeks postpartum.

21. _____ Weight loss of 30 lb

22. _____ Abdominal musculature somewhat lax

23. _____ Striae pink and readily apparent

24. _____ Nonbreastfeeding mother: breasts firm to the touch

25. _____ Normal bowel elimination pattern

26. _____ Lochia serosa, scant

27. _____ Fundus not palpable above symphysis

28. During a home visit, you assess a new mother for signs of bonding with her infant. List at least five signs that might indicate a failure to bond.

    a.

    b.

c.

d.

e.

SUPPORT FOR THE BREASTFEEDING MOTHER

29. **Nursing Care Plan in Action:** For the following case scenario, focus on the pertinent data, formulate one appropriate nursing diagnosis, and complete all components of the nursing care plan.

    Case Scenario: Natalie is breastfeeding for the first time. She tells you that breastfeeding has been going well but she never dreamed it would hurt so much to breastfeed. No one ever said it would hurt. Upon assessing her breasts you note slightly reddened nipples. When Natalie breastfeeds her baby, she has a look of anticipated pain as the baby latches on and grimaces as her baby suckles.

    Collaborative problems:

    Nursing diagnosis:

    Defining characteristics:

Goal/Evaluation Criteria	Nursing Activities	Evaluation of Goal
Client will:	Assessments:	

(continued)

Goal/Evaluation Criteria	Nursing Activities	Evaluation of Goal
	Interventions:	

Match the following descriptions with the appropriate breastfeeding problem.

30. _____ Cracked nipples

31. _____ Plugged ducts

32. _____ Engorgement

33. _____ Inverted nipples

34. _____ Nipple soreness

a. Caused by improper positioning and improper latch-on

b. Fissures appear on nipple(s)

c. Nipples fail to protrude, or point toward chest wall

d. Area of tenderness or lumpiness

e. Breasts are hard, painful, and warm, and appear taut and shiny

CHAPTER 20

THE POSTPARTAL FAMILY AT RISK

The emotional support and teaching a postpartal nurse provides cannot be overemphasized, nor can the nurse's responsibility to carefully monitor the mother's physical status. Complications do sometimes develop in the birthing center or at home during the postpartal period, but their severity may often be ameliorated by early detection and interaction.

This chapter corresponds to Chapter 38 in the eighth edition of *Olds' Maternal-Newborn Nursing & Women's Health Across the Lifespan.*

POSTPARTAL HEMORRHAGE

1. Postpartal hemorrhage may be classified as early or late. Describe the time of onset and primary cause(s) of each.

   a. Early

   b. Late

Joan Taranta, a 33-year-old gravida 3 para 3, is recovering following the birth of twin boys. Her labor lasted 2½ hours.

2. Identify two factors that predispose Joan to early postpartal hemorrhage.

   a.

   b.

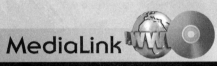

MediaLink

http://www.prenhall.com/davidson

Additional resources for this content can be found on the Student DVD-ROM accompanying the eighth edition of *Olds' Maternal-Newborn Nursing & Women's Health Across the Lifespan,* and on the Companion Website at http://www.prenhall.com/davidson. Click on the text chapter number(s) listed for this content to select the appropriate activities.

Prentice Hall Nursing MediaLink DVD-ROM
- Audio Glossary
- NCLEX Review

Companion Website
- Additional NCLEX Review
- Case Study: Postpartal Client with Thromboembolic Disease
- Care Plan Activity: Postpartal Perineal Pain

3. During your assessment of Joan, what three findings would indicate possible early postpartal hemorrhage?

   a.

   b.

   c.

4. The nurse finds Joan's uterus to be boggy, high, and deviated to the right. The most appropriate nursing action is to

   a. have Joan void and then reevaluate the fundus.

   b. massage the uterus and reevaluate in 30 minutes.

   c. notify the physician.

   d. place Joan on a pad count.

5. What do you consider the two highest priorities in planning your care of Joan?

6. What additional nursing interventions should be initiated for Joan as she demonstrates signs of postpartal hemorrhage?

7. **Critical Thinking in Practice:** The following action sequence is designed to help you think through basic clinical problems (see page 221).

   You are taking care of Mrs. Carrie Spencer, age 24, gravida 1 para 1, on the mother-baby unit. She is 8 hours postbirth of an 8 lb, 2 oz baby girl. As you are carrying out her postpartal assessments, she complains of tenderness and pain in her perineal area. She says, "My stitches hurt; it feels as if they are tearing apart."

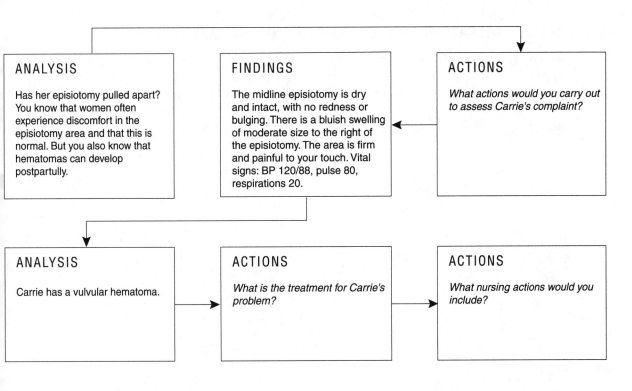

ANALYSIS

Has her episiotomy pulled apart? You know that women often experience discomfort in the episiotomy area and that this is normal. But you also know that hematomas can develop postpartully.

FINDINGS

The midline episiotomy is dry and intact, with no redness or bulging. There is a bluish swelling of moderate size to the right of the episiotomy. The area is firm and painful to your touch. Vital signs: BP 120/88, pulse 80, respirations 20.

ACTIONS

What actions would you carry out to assess Carrie's complaint?

ANALYSIS

Carrie has a vulvular hematoma.

ACTIONS

What is the treatment for Carrie's problem?

ACTIONS

What nursing actions would you include?

REFLECTIONS

Have you provided care for a woman experiencing bleeding in the immediate postpartal period? What concerns did she express? Describe the experience.

_____

_____

_____

_____

_____

_____

_____

LATE POSTPARTAL HEMORRHAGE/SUBINVOLUTION

Mrs. Gloria Brown, a breastfeeding mother, gave birth to an 8 lb, 11 1/2 oz baby boy, Vincent, vaginally after Pitocin augmentation. She has been home for 2 weeks and calls the office. She tells the Ob/Gyn nurse practitioner that she is concerned because her flow has increased and is red but not foul smelling.

8. Identify nursing assessments that might lead you to suspect subinvolution.

9. Identify three nursing interventions to meet Mrs. Brown's needs.

REPRODUCTIVE TRACT OR WOUND INFECTIONS

10. The clinical manifestations of a localized infection of the episiotomy would include

    a. approximation of the skin edges of the episiotomy.

    b. client complaint of severe discomfort in the perineum and an oral temperature of 99.8F (37.7C).

    c. reddened, bruised tissue.

    d. reddened, edematous tissue with yellowish discharge.

Felipe and Celestina just had their third baby by cesarean birth.

11. The nurse's assessment of Celestina reveals an elevation in her temperature, chills, nausea, and increased pain. The nurse notifies the primary physician and receives the following orders: ampicillin 500 mg IV every 6 hours; culture and sensitivity of lochia; ultrasound of the pelvis; and a chest x-ray. Which order should the nurse carry out first?

    a. Chest x-ray

    b. Culture of lochia

    c. IV antibiotic

    d. Ultrasound

12. Celestina's incision has become infected, and she has been placed in intensive care. Because the baby can no longer room in, how can the nurse promote bonding between Celestina and her infant?

    a. Assure Celestina she will be in intensive care only a short time.

    b. Encourage Celestina to use the time away from the baby to rest so she will recover faster.

    c. Have Felipe visit the baby more often.

    d. Provide a picture of the baby for Celestina.

13. Complete the following chart on puerperal infection:

Component	Localized Infection (Episiotomy and/or Laceration)	Metritis (Endometritis)	Pelvic Cellulitis (Parametritis)
Tissues involved			
Clinical manifestations			
Interventions			
Potential complications			

14. Identify evaluative outcome criteria findings that indicate your interventions/treatments of the puerperal infection have been effective.

15. What home care instructions about puerperal infections would you give a mother?

OVERDISTENTION OF BLADDER

16. **Critical Thinking Challenge:** The following situation has been included to challenge your critical thinking. Read the situation, answer the question "yes" or "no," and give your rationale (see page 224).

    Jeanne McGuire, age 34, gravida 3 para 3, gave birth to twin boys vaginally with regional anesthesia 12 hours ago and you are now responsible for her care. She complains of cramping when the uterus attempts to contract. Your assessment reveals a uterus one fingerbreadth above the umbilicus and displaced to the right, and increased vaginal bleeding.

Is Mrs. McGuire a candidate for bladder distention?

Yes _____   No _____

Explain your answer:

POSTPARTAL CYSTITIS

17. Identify appropriate self-care measures to prevent postpartal cystitis.

MASTITIS

One week after her discharge, Yaeko Manning, a 23-year-old, gravida 1 para 1 breastfeeding mother, develops mastitis.

18. List two factors that contribute to the development of mastitis.

    a.

    b.

19. Identify four clinical manifestations of mastitis that Yaeko may exhibit.

    a.

    b.

    c.

    d.

Two nursing diagnoses that may apply to Yaeko are **Acute Pain related to inflammation and swelling of breast tissue and Health-Seeking Behavior related to lack of information about appropriate breastfeeding techniques.**

20. Based on these possible nursing diagnoses, describe the interventions that Yaeko or you may institute.

THROMBOEMBOLIC DISEASES

21. Identify the physiologic changes of pregnancy and predisposing factors that increase a woman's susceptibility to blood clot formation during the postpartal period.

22. Identify three interventions useful in preventing the development of thrombophlebitis during the postpartal period.

    a.

    b.

    c.

Match the following descriptive statements with the correct thromboembolic disease.

23. _____ Clotting process involving the saphenous vein system

24. _____ More frequently seen in women with history of thrombosis

25. _____ Usually appears about third or fourth postpartal day

26. _____ Sudden onset of sweating, pallor, dyspnea, and chest pain

27. _____ Prompt intervention with heparin, oxygen, and lidocaine as needed

28. _____ Edema of ankle and leg; low-grade fever and positive Homans' sign

29. _____ Treatment primarily involves IV heparin and bed rest

30. _____ Management principally involves leg elevation, moist packs, bed rest, and elastic support stockings

a. Superficial thrombophlebitis

b. Deep vein thrombosis (DVT)

c. Pulmonary embolism

31. Lenda Cortez has developed thrombophlebitis and is receiving heparin intravenously. It will be important to watch her for signs of overdose, which include

   a. epistaxis, hematuria, and dysuria.

   b. dysuria.

   c. hematuria, ecchymosis, and epistaxis.

   d. hematuria, ecchymosis, and vertigo.

32. The antagonist of heparin is _____.

33. A positive Homans' sign is indicated by a complaint of pain in

   a. the foot when the client stands.

   b. the leg when the foot is dorsiflexed while the knee is held flat.

   c. the leg when the knee is flexed and the foot is extended.

   d. the leg when the knee is held flat and the foot is rotated.

34. What education for self-care at home should be given to a woman receiving warfarin (Coumadin)?

POSTPARTAL MOOD DISORDERS

It is the third postpartal day for Bonnie Sumpter, an 18-year-old primipara. She is single and is keeping her baby. The nurse makes a home visit and expresses concern that Bonnie may not be bonding appropriately with her infant.

35. Identify four feelings or behaviors that might indicate "postpartum blues."

    a.

    b.

    c.

    d.

EPILOGUE

By now you are probably almost finished with your maternity nursing rotation. We hope this workbook has helped you focus your study so that you are more comfortable in relating your knowledge of theory to your clinical practice. We believe that in this way you will be better nurses, and that the childbearing families for whom you are responsible will receive better care.

Answer Key

Chapter 1

1. Answers include the following: partner and family in the labor room with the laboring woman; newborns in the room with their mothers during the postpartum period; siblings allowed to visit the maternity unit; fathers able to be actively involved in the labor and birth process; availability of family choices about the labor and birth (place of birth, primary caregiver, birth-related experiences); shortened length of stay for the new mother and her infant.

2. (a) The professional nurse has graduated from a basic, accredited program in nursing, has successfully passed the NCLEX nursing examination, and is licensed as a registered nurse; (b) the CNS has a master's degree and specialized knowledge and competence in a specific clinical area; (c) the NP has received specialized education in a master's degree program or certificate program and can function in an advanced practice role; (d) the CNM is educated as both a nurse and a midwife and is certified by the American College of Nurse-Midwives.

3. b

4. health promotion, illness prevention, and individual responsibility

5. community-based

6. (a) Provides opportunity for additional support and teaching following discharge from an acute care setting; (b) enables people to remain at home with conditions that formerly would have required hospitalization.

7. See text, pp. 9–10.

8. (a) The information must be clearly and concisely presented in a way that is understandable to the client; (b) it must include information on the risks and benefits, the probability of success, and significant treatment alternatives; (c) it must include information on the consequences of receiving no treatment or procedure; and (d) the client must be told of the right to refuse a specific treatment or procedure without fear that all support or care will be withdrawn.

9. (a) Number of live births per 1000 people; (b) number of deaths of infants under 1 year of age per 1000 live births in a given population; (c) number of deaths of infants less than 28 days of age per 1000 live births; (d) number of deaths from any cause during the pregnancy cycle (including the 42-day postpartal period) per 100,000 live births.

10. Answers include the following: increased use of hospitals and specialized healthcare personnel by maternity clients; improved high-risk care for mothers and infants; prevention and control of infection with antibiotics and improved techniques; availability of blood and blood products for transfusions; lowered rates of anesthesia-related deaths.

11. d

12. Evidence-based practice is a process of thoughtful analysis that uses forms of evidence such as statistical data, research findings, quality measures, risk management measures, and information from support services to guide problem solving and decision making.

13. A family is defined traditionally as individuals joined together by marriage, blood, adoption, or residence in the same household. More broadly a family includes individuals who are joined together by ties of emotional closeness and sharing and who consider themselves part of a family.

14. a

15. culture

16. See text, pp. 43–44.

17. A complementary therapy is an adjunct to conventional medical treatment. It has been through rigorous scientific testing that shows that it has some reliability. An alternative therapy has not undergone rigorous scientific testing in the United States, although it might have been

thoroughly tested in other countries. Alternative therapies are sometimes considered less "mainstream."

18. j   19. g   20. f   21. e   22. i
23. a   24. h   25. d   26. b

Chapter 2

1. Women's health is a concept that considers a woman and her healthcare needs holistically within the context of her life and the factors that influence her health status. These include her physical, mental, and spiritual status, the impact of family and culture, and so forth.

2. b   3. a   4. c   5. e   6. f   7. d

8. See text, pp. 73–74.

9. Your text provides a complete list for you. Many of the considerations—such as eating a nutritious, balanced diet, maintaining normal weight for height (no fad dieting), performing regular aerobic exercise and weight training several times a week, getting adequate sleep, avoiding smoking and/or stopping smoking, consuming alcohol in moderation, managing stress effectively, and keeping health maintenance activities current—are well recognized. However, did you also think about the other factors related to lifestyle such as developing enjoyable hobbies and leisure activities, developing an inner life, and fostering bonds of affection and support with family and friends? Those activities are equally important in helping shape a healthy life.

10. The period of time before menopause during which the woman moves from normal ovulatory cycles to cessation of menses.

11. (a) decreasing ovarian function, (b) unstable endocrine physiology, (c) highly variable, unpredictable hormone profiles.

12. Mrs. Sanchez might benefit from information about the following self-care measures: the use of a fan and/or the increased intake of cool liquids for the hot flashes, continued calcium supplementation, and the use of water-soluble jelly during intercourse to counteract the dryness associated with vaginal atrophy (increased frequency of intercourse will also maintain some elasticity in the vagina if this is an area of concern for her). It may also be of value to discuss other physical and emotional responses that may occur in menopause.

13. If you answered "yes," you are correct. Congratulations. Ms. Swenson has several factors that place her at risk for osteoporosis, including early onset of menopause, fair complexion, slender build, and a history of smoking.

14. (a) progestin, (b) endometrial cancer

15. b   16. b   17. a   18. b   19. a   20. a

21. (a) 6 (b) 6

22. IUDs are recommended for women who have given birth to a child and who are in a mutually monogamous sexual relationship. Until Marcella is sure that the relationship will be long term and that the man is not sexually active with multiple partners, she is safer choosing another method of contraception. Regardless of the method she chooses, she should insist that her partner use a condom.

23. (a) vasectomy, (b) tubal ligation

24. d

25. (a) transdermal, (b) weekly, (c) 1 week

26. (a) 21, (b) 7

27. Lunelle, a combined contraceptive, contains both estrogen and a progestin. Depo-Provera is a progesterone-only contraceptive.

28. (a) unprotected intercourse, (b) possible contraceptive failure, (c) 72

29. (a) 7, (b) mifepristone, (c) misoprostol

30. (a) stomach pain, (b) weakness, (c) nausea, (d) vomiting or diarrhea

31. She should contact her caregiver immediately.

Chapter 3

1. c   2. a   3. b   4. a
5. d   6. c   7. a   8. b

9. *Actions:* In making your assessment it would be helpful to ask Nita whether she has noticed any change in her vaginal discharge. If she has, ask her to describe it. Because of the relationship between antibiotic therapy and monilial infection, you would ask whether she had been on antibiotics for any reason. It is always useful to ask clients whether they attribute the symptoms to anything. You may gain useful information about the condition or information about the client's perceptions.

Analysis: Based on the information obtained, you suspect that Nita has vulvovaginal candidiasis (VVC).

Actions: You tell Nita that, based on her symptoms, you suspect that she may have a yeast infection called vulvovaginal candidiasis. You point out that sometimes when women take antibiotics to destroy a bacterial infection, the antibiotics also destroy the normal, good bacteria found in a woman's vagina. When this happens, other organisms, especially yeast, may grow unchecked. You tell Nita that you will report your findings to the nurse practitioner (NP). You point out that the NP will probably do a vaginal examination and a test to confirm the infection type.

Actions: You would briefly describe Nita's symptoms and the appearance of her vaginal discharge and report the recent antibiotic therapy. You would say that you suspect that Nita might have VVC and ask the NP if she or he planned to do a vaginal examination and wet prep.

Analysis: Congratulations! Your analysis of the data was accurate. Hyphae and spores indicate VVC. Give yourself a pat on the back, too, for working in a collegial fashion with the NP.

10. (a) venereal warts or genital warts, (b) human papilloma virus, (c) cervical dysplasia or cervical cancer

11. d

12. Warn Mica that she and her partner should avoid drinking alcohol while taking metronidazole because the combination has an effect similar to that of alcohol and Antabuse, including abdominal pain, flushing, and tremors.

13. infertility

14. See text, pp. 121–123.

15. All women have breasts that vary slightly in size and contour, but inspection helps a woman know her own breasts so that she can recognize changes. Changes in the way her breasts move or point as she moves them through a variety of positions can be significant. Moving the arms varies the pull on the skin and muscle of the chest so that masses or changes that are not visible in one position may become evident in another position.

16. See text, pp. 127–130.

17. d 18. d 19. a 20. e

21. You would probably mention simple practices such as limiting sodium intake and wearing a supportive bra. For more severe discomfort, the woman may ask her caregiver for a prescription for a mild diuretic and might also use an over-the-counter analgesic. Even though controversy exists about the effectiveness of limiting methylxanthines (found in caffeine products), it can't hurt, and many women feel it is helpful. If you give the woman this information, she can then choose whether she wishes to try it. Other

approaches include the use of thiamine and vitamin E. Use this time to stress the importance of monthly breast self-examination, annual examinations by her healthcare provider, and regular mammograms as recommended by her healthcare provider.

22. (a) pelvic pain, (b) dyspareunia, (c) abnormal uterine bleeding

23. We hope you would discuss her medication in detail with her. It is important to review the purpose of the medication and possible side effects. You should also be certain that she clearly understands the dosage and administration schedule. In many instances women take danazol for a specified period of time (from 3 to 8 months or longer), depending on the severity of the disease and the presence of palpable lesions. If she is scheduled to return for reevaluation at specified times, it is important that she understand the purpose and significance of these evaluations. Answer any questions she might have and give her an opportunity to voice any concerns about the therapy. If this medication is prescribed frequently in your office, you may want to develop a handout on it for clients to refer to when they are at home.

24. b

25. Your recommendations should include the following: Women with a history of TSS should *never* use tampons; others should avoid prolonged use of tampons, change tampons every 3–6 hours, avoid superabsorbent tampons, avoid overnight use of tampons, alternate tampons with sanitary napkins or minipads, and avoid tampon use for 6–8 weeks after childbirth. In addition, women should avoid leaving diaphragms or cervical caps in place for extended periods of time and never use them postpartally or when menstruating. They should also be aware of the signs of TSS.

26. c 27. b 28. d

29. At age 18 or when they become sexually active, whichever occurs first.

30. dysfunctional uterine bleeding (DUB)

31. (a) cystocele, (b) rectocele

32. (a) Total abdominal hysterectomy and bilateral salpingo-oophorectomy, (b) Through an abdominal incision, the uterus, both ovaries, and both fallopian tubes are removed.

33. Female-headed household and minority race

34. See text, pp. 158–159.

35. See text, p. 160.

36. Occupational Safety and Health Administration

37. OSHA is responsible for creating and enforcing workplace health and safety regulations.

38. National Institute for Occupational Safety and Health

39. NIOSH is primarily a research agency, but it also disseminates information on preventing workplace injury and illness, provides training to occupational safety and health professionals, and investigates potentially hazardous working situations when requested by employers or employees.

40. Answers may include the following: women have a longer life expectancy; older women tend to have less educational preparation than older men; many women are economically dependent on men and may have intermittent or nonexistent employment histories; women typically earn less than men; women often work in jobs without pension benefits or only limited benefits; women generally have more family caregiving responsibilities than older men; women, more often than men, feel the impact of public policies and programs that place undue financial pressures on them.

41. Any deliberate action or lack of action that causes harm to an elderly person.

42. Psychologic abuse, physical abuse, neglect (by self or caregiver), financial abuse, and abandonment

43. See text, pp. 170–172.

44. Methods used to exert power and control by one individual over another in an adult intimate relationship. Because 95% of the victims are women, this is also termed *female partner abuse*.

45. one; three

46. (a) Within the last year, have you been hit, slapped, kicked, choked, or otherwise physically hurt by someone? (b) Within the last year has anyone forced you to have sex? (c) Are you afraid of anyone at home or an ex-partner?

47. See text, p. 187.

48. c   49. a   50. b   51. d

52. See text, p. 193.

Chapter 4

1. c   2. b   3. a   4. f   5. d   6. e

7. See Figure 10–4.

8. The vagina serves as a passageway for sperm, fetal birth, and the products of menstruation. It protects against trauma from sexual intercourse and infection.

9. Factors that can destroy the self-cleansing ability of the vagina include antibiotic therapy, douching, and use of perineal sprays or deodorants.

10. (a) isthmus of fallopian tube, (b) uterine cavity, (c) uterine body, (d) endometrium, (e) myometrium, (f) internal os, (g) isthmus, (h) cervix, (i) vagina

11. b

12. The endometrium produces a thin, watery, alkaline secretion that helps sperm travel to the fallopian tubes; it nourishes the developing embryo before implantation.

13. (a) lubricates vaginal canal, (b) acts as a bacteriostatic action, (c) provides an alkaline environment to protect sperm from the acidic vagina

14. b   15. d

16. The fallopian tubes provide transport for the ovum from the ovary to the uterus (which takes 72–96 hours); a site for fertilization; and a warm, moist, nourishing environment for the ovum and zygote.

17. See text, pp. 212–213.

18. See text, p. 213.

19. The ovaries secrete estrogen and progesterone and are responsible for ovulation.

20. See text, pp. 211–212.

21. See Figure 10–12.

22. (a) Portion above pelvic brim or linea terminalis; supports the pregnant uterus; directs the presenting fetal part into true pelvis below.

(b) Lies below the linea terminalis; its shape and size determine the adequacy of the birth passage.

(c) Upper border of true pelvis; usually rounded; determines whether engagement can occur.

(d) Lower border of the true pelvis; if too narrow the baby's head may be pushed backward, making extension difficult and causing shoulder dystocia for large babies.

23. (a) false pelvis, (b) true pelvis, (c) pelvic inlet, (d) pelvic outlet (see Figure 10–13)

24. See Figure 10–16.

25. The tubercles of Montgomery secrete a fatty substance that helps lubricate and protect the breasts.

26. a

27. (a) ovarian, (b) menstrual

28. See text, pp. 219–221.

29. c   30. a

31. *Follicular phase:* under the influence of FSH, the graafian follicle matures; LH assists the oocyte in rupturing out of the ovary around day 14.

Luteal phase: after rupture, the corpus luteum (CL) forms; if fertilization does not occur, the CL degenerates and progesterone and estrogen decrease, which results in menses.

32. See text, pp. 222–223.

33. See Figure 10–18.

34. a

35. (a) penis, (b) epididymides, (c) vas deferens, (d) testes, (e) testis, (f) Leydig's cells, (g) seminiferous tubules, (h) Sertoli's, (i) seminal vesicles, (j) ejaculatory duct, (k) prostate, (l) seminal fluid, (m) bulbourethral (Cowper's)

36. (a) female reproductive cycle, (b) follicle-stimulating hormone, (c) gonadotropin-releasing hormone, (d) luteinizing hormone

Chapter 5

1. *Mitosis:* Process to reproduce all body cells so that each cell is an exact replica of the original cell.

   Meiosis: A two-stage division process that ends with each cell having only half the number (23) of chromosomes of other body cells; process of replication for ovum and sperm only.

2. (a) 23, (b) 46

3. (a) 12–24, (b) 24

4. c   5. b

6. See text, pp. 236–237.

7. (a) XY, (b) male

8. a   9. a   10. c   11. d   12. e   13. b

14. (a) 7, (b) 9; Trophoblasts attach themselves to the endometrium for nourishment; the blastocyst burrows beneath the uterine lining, which then thickens below the blastocyst; and the trophoblastic cells grow into the lining and form villi.

15. b   16. c

17. (a) chorion, (b) amnion

18. (a) decidua vera, (b) decidua basalis, (c) chorion, (d) amnion, (e) decidua capsularis

19. a, b, d   20. c

21. (a) 1, (b) 2, (c) Wharton's jelly, (d) prevent compression of the umbilical cord in utero

22. The maternal side appears red and fleshlike and is made up of the decidua basalis and its circulation. The fetal side appears shiny and gray and consists of the chorionic villi and their circulation; the placenta at term weighs 400 to 600 g, and its diameter is 15 to 20 cm (5.9 to 7.9 in.).

23. See text, p. 246.

24. Answers may include the following functions: metabolic, transport, endocrine, immunologic.

25. The significant observations that you would want to make about the placenta would include determining the presence of all cotyledons, the presence of large infarcts or clots in the placenta, and the site of the umbilical insertion on the placenta. These observations will give you clues to potential problems for the newborn. The absence of cotyledons would indicate a need to have the clinician check the mother for retained placental fragments that could cause postpartum hemorrhage later.

26. (a) The embryonic stage starts on day 15 and continues until approximately the eighth week or until the embryo reaches a crown-rump (C-R) length of 3 cm or 1.2 in. (b) By the end of the eighth week, every organ system and external structures are present.

27. oxygenated, to; deoxygenated, from

28. (a) ductus arteriosus, (b) foramen ovale, (c) inferior vena cava, (d) ductus venosus, (e) umbilical vein, (f) umbilical arteries

29. Fetal circulation differs significantly from infant and adult circulation in that the fetus's oxygenated blood originates from the placenta and flows into the right atrium. It then moves through the foramen ovale (because of the low resistance on the left side of the fetal heart) and out the aorta to provide the head and upper body with highly oxygenated blood. Very little oxygenated blood flows into the lungs because they are collapsed and offer a high resistance to blood flow. The blood that goes through the pulmonary artery is shunted into the aorta through the ductus arteriosus, bypassing the lungs to supply the rest of the body. See text Chapter 28 for natal (postbirth) circulation.

30. d

31. (a) 16 weeks; (b) 13.5 cm C–R, 15 cm C–H, 200 g; (c) 20 weeks; (d) 4 weeks; (e) 16 weeks; (f) Yes, eyes close at the 10th week and then reopen about the 28th week of gestation.

32. Many factors can influence the development of the embryo or fetus. Significant factors include the quality of the sperm or ova, teratogenic agents such as drugs, hyperthermia, and maternal nutrition. Others you might have identified are any of the complications of pregnancy, such as maternal diabetes, hypertension, or viral infections.

33. a, b

34. (a) Lack of conception despite unprotected sexual intercourse for at least 12 months; (b) Difficulty in conceiving because both partners have reduced fertility.

35. You could discuss self-care actions that can support fertility, for example: avoiding douching and artificial lubricants that alter vaginal pH and adopting positions during intercourse that support retention of sperm. For further self-care measures, see Table 12–2 in text.

36. See text, pp. 268–269.

37. a   38. d   39. c   40. b   41. f

42. e   43. g

44. See text, p. 268, Table 12–5.

45. a   46. a, b, c

47. (a) A combination of FSH and LH administered IM to stimulate follicular development; monitor serum estradiol levels and ultrasound. (b) Used to treat hyperprolactimia; side effects may include nausea, diarrhea, dizziness, headaches.

48. a

49. See text, pp. 273–277.

50. A possible nursing diagnosis that would apply is **Disturbance in Self-Esteem related to infertility.** This diagnosis depends on how successful the couple is in adjusting to the loss of the ability to conceive a child. Other nursing diagnoses that might apply are **Ineffective Individual (or Family) Coping related to inability to accept infertility, or Grieving related to loss of fertility** if the couple has made the decision to accept their childless status. Defining characteristics that are present include negative body image (". . . my body can't do what it should"), low self-esteem (expressed feelings of failure), and failure in role performance ("I am such a failure as a woman").

51. a

52. karyotype

53. Each child has a 50% chance of developing Huntington chorea. For diagram, see Figure 12–19 in text.

54. c. See Figure 12–20 in text.

55. See text, pp. 273, 289, Developing Cultural Competence.

56. See Figure 12–24. We hope you have learned interesting and helpful information about your family to facilitate your self-care.

57. (a) amniotic fluid, (b) basal body temperature, (c) human chorionic gonadotropin, (d) human chorionic somatomammotropin, (e) human menopausal gonadotropin, (f) human placental lactogen

Chapter 6

1. Answers may include the following: Both Gretta and her partner should have a physical examination and should act to correct any identified problems such as infection or hypertension. If she is nonimmune to rubella, she should consider receiving the vaccine and then waiting to conceive. Gretta should also discontinue birth control pills at least 3 months before conceiving; strengthen healthful behaviors such as stress reduction, regular exercise, and healthy eating; and reduce or eliminate behaviors that are known to have adverse affects on pregnancy and fetal growth, such as smoking cigarettes or cigars, drinking alcoholic drinks, and using illegal drugs. If Gretta's partner smokes, uses alcohol, or takes illegal drugs, it will be helpful for him to change these behaviors too.

2. A birth plan is a document formulated by the childbearing couple (or the pregnant woman alone if the father is not involved) that identifies the decisions they have made regarding all aspects of their childbirth experience.

3. Answers may include the following: type of care provider, desired birth setting, participation in prenatal classes, method of childbirth preparation, partner's degree of involvement in the labor and birth, presence of other family members at the birth, use of other labor support such as a doula, use of analgesia or anesthesia, postpartum care, newborn care.

4. See text, pp. 307–308.

5. c.

6. The uterus, fetus, and placenta require additional blood flow. By the end of pregnancy, one sixth of the total maternal blood volume is found in the vascular system of the uterus.

7. (a) Chadwick's, (b) Goodell's, (c) Hegar's

8. d

9. The function of the mucous plug is to prevent the ascent of organisms from the vaginal tract into the uterus.

10. stop

11. d

12. Acid pH helps prevent bacterial infections; however, it favors the growth of yeast organisms.

13. (a) increase in size, (b) areolas darken, (c) Montgomery's tubercles become more pronounced and enlarged

14. Nasal stuffiness and epistaxis occur because of estrogen-induced edema and vascular congestion of the nasal mucosa.

15. D   16. I   17. I   18. D   19. I   20. D

21. (a) supine hypotensive, (b) aortocaval, (c) vena caval

22. a

23. (a) The relaxed cardiac sphincter and pressure from the enlarging uterus on the stomach promote reflux of gastric acid secretions into the lower esophagus. (b) Hemorrhoids may be related to constipation and pressure on vessels below the level of the uterus. (c) The pressure of the enlarging uterus on the bladder in the first and third trimesters increases urinary frequency.

24. b   25. c   26. d   27. b   28. a

29. We are assuming you would take the time to find out if the comments bothered the woman and how she perceives her body image during pregnancy. In answer to her specific questions, you can point out that her stomach-first walk occurs because the weight and size of her growing uterus cause her center of gravity to change. To compensate, pregnant women tend to exaggerate the lumbar curve, which may result in backache. Because hormonal effects produce softening of the pelvic joints, the woman's walk assumes a more "waddling" appearance. This may be made more noticeable because many pregnant women also tend to walk with their feet farther apart to help maintain balance.

30. (a) Stimulates estrogen and progesterone production by the corpus luteum until the placenta is sufficiently developed; (b) stimulates uterine development and development of the ductal system of the breasts for lactation; (c) helps maintain pregnancy; also promotes development of the acini and lobules of the breasts for lactation; (d) decreases maternal metabolism of glucose to favor fetal growth and increases amount of circulating free fatty acids for maternal metabolic needs; (e) inhibits uterine activity and helps remodel collagen.

31. See text, pp. 320–321.

32. Prostaglandins may maintain reduced placental vascular resistance. They may also play a role in the initiation of labor.

33. 25 to 35 lb (11.5 to 16 kg)

34. (a) 3.5 to 5 lb (1.6 to 2.3 kg); (b) and (c) 12 to 15 lb (5.5 to 6.8 kg)

35. S   36. O   37. D   38. S   39. O

40. S   41. O   42. S   43. D   44. O

45. Subjective signs are symptoms the woman experiences and reports; they may have causes other than pregnancy. Objective signs may be perceived by an examiner; they may have causes other than pregnancy. Diagnostic signs are perceived by an examiner and may only be caused by pregnancy.

46. See text, p. 324.

47. A positive pregnancy test may be caused by factors other than pregnancy, such as choriocarcinoma, hydatidiform mole, or menopause.

48. c

49. See text, pp. 326–330.

50. The effects of pregnancy on a woman's body image are greatly influenced by her feelings about her pregnancy and by cultural, physiologic, psychosocial, and interpersonal factors. Some women experience the "glow of pregnancy" in the second trimester when they begin wearing maternity clothes. In the last weeks of pregnancy, a woman may feel constantly tired and misshapen and may, as a result, have a negative body image. You are on the right track if you recognized that a variety of factors influence body image. Although there is no one correct answer, certain types of responses occur frequently.

51. Rubin (1984) identified the following psychologic tasks of the pregnant woman: (a) Ensuring safe passage through pregnancy, labor, and birth. The woman's concern for herself and her unborn child leads her to select a caregiver she trusts and to seek information about birth from classes, friends, and literature. She becomes more concerned about safety—both hers and her partner's. (b) Seeking acceptance of this child by others. The woman is concerned about her family's acceptance of the child, but her partner's reaction and acceptance are of primary importance to her successful completion of her developmental tasks. She also works to ensure the acceptance of the unborn child by other children in the family. The woman subtly alters her secondary network of friends as necessary to meet the demands of her pregnancy. (c) Seeking commitment and acceptance of self as mother to the infant—"binding-in." With quickening, the mother begins to develop bonds of attachment to the child and commits herself to the child's welfare. (d) Learning to give of self on behalf of child. The woman begins to develop a capacity for self-denial and delayed personal gratification to meet the needs of another. Baby showers and gifts increase the mother's self-esteem while helping her accept the separateness and needs of her coming child.

52. b

53. We hope you would tell your friend that, even in the most desired pregnancy, feelings of ambivalence are normal. Role changes, physical changes, altered relationships, added financial responsibilities, and attitudes about parenting and values all affect a woman's—indeed a couple's—response to pregnancy.

54. See text, pp. 330–331.

55. Traditionally, *couvade* referred to the male's observance of certain rites and rituals as part of his transition to fatherhood. Today, the term is used to describe the unintentional development of physical symptoms such as fatigue, headache, or difficulty sleeping by the partner of the pregnant woman.

56. See text, pp. 331–333.

57. Initially, it may be difficult for a nurse to recognize and accept cultural diversity. To do so, the nurse needs to develop cultural competency. The following points may help a nurse become more effective in caring for people from different cultures: (a) People have a tendency to project their own cultural responses onto people from another culture, and thus they assume that the person is acting from similar motives or values. Often this is not correct and leads to misunderstanding. For example, a nurse who highly values promptness may view a client's lateness as a personal insult when, in reality, the client is much less time oriented and doesn't place the same value on promptness. (b) Unless there is a clear health contraindication to a particular cultural practice, nurses should avoid interfering in a client's health practices. If the client's beliefs are potentially harmful, the nurse can try to persuade the woman to change. However, if the woman refuses to change, the nurse must accept the woman's right to make her own health choices. (c) Before considering any intervention, the nurse should try to determine the impact of traditional practices on the planned intervention. (d) Practices and beliefs vary not only from one culture to another but also within a culture. These variations are often related to social and economic factors such as class, income, and education. (e) Nurses often find it helpful to begin developing cultural awareness by learning some of the basic beliefs and practices of minority cultures in their area. (f) Foster an attitude of respect for and cooperation with alternative healers and caregivers whenever possible. (g) Provide for the services of an interpreter if language barriers exist. (h) Learn the language (or at least several key phrases) of at least one of the cultural groups with whom you interact.

If you included some of these ideas, you are well on your way to developing cultural sensitivity. This is a challenging area for healthcare providers. We hope you can become comfortable working with people from other cultures.

58. (a) human chorionic gonadotropin, (b) human placental lactogen

Chapter 7

1. The initial client history is important in determining the status of the woman's health before the onset of pregnancy. It helps caregivers identify factors that might place the woman at risk during her pregnancy.

2. d   3. a   4. b   5. f   6. c

7. Roya is a gravida 4, para 2, ab 1, living children 2.

8. (a) Yolanda is a gravida 3, para 2, ab 0, living children 1. If you recorded this differently, was it because you forgot that a stillborn infant would be considered viable at 36 weeks and would therefore count as a para? (b) Using the detailed approach, Yolanda would be a gravida 3, para 1101 Yolanda's stillborn infant would be considered a preterm birth.

9. Taking an obstetric health history should help you focus on the information that is pertinent to high-quality maternity care. You should be able to identify a reason for each of the questions asked. You should also be able to identify information that may place a client in the high-risk category. In addition to such obvious problems as preexisting medical conditions, think about maternal age, weight, occupation, and previous obstetric history; family history of disorders; marital status and support system; smoking and alcohol consumption; and so on. Once you begin to recognize risk factors, you will be better able to plan for appropriate antepartal care.

10. N   11. A   12. A   13. N   14. N

15. Risk factors are any findings that suggest the pregnancy may have a negative outcome.

16. Answers may include the following: use of addicting drugs; preexisting medical disorders such as diabetes, heart condition, or thyroid disorder; maternal anemia; excessive alcohol consumption; history of habitual spontaneous abortion; multiple gestation; spontaneous premature rupture of the membranes.

17. Jenny's initial obstetric examination focuses on inspection, auscultation, and palpation of the abdomen; determination of the adequacy of the pelvis; and vaginal examination.

18. Fundal height is measured in centimeters after the woman has voided. She should lie in the same position each time (generally supine). The zero line of the tape measure is placed on the superior border of the symphysis pubis, and the tape is stretched over the midline of the woman's abdomen to the top of the fundus (see text, Figure 15–4, p. 352).

19. (a) Between 22 to 24 weeks and 34 weeks, fundal height in centimeters generally correlates with weeks of gestation; (b) slightly above the symphysis pubis; (c) at the umbilicus (see text, Figure 14–6, p. 324).

20. On average, by 10 to 12 weeks' gestation.

21. lithotomy

22. The initial pelvic examination should include a Pap smear and any other pertinent cultures or smears; visual inspection of the external genitalia, vagina, and cervix; and a bimanual examination.

23. A diagonal conjugate of 9 cm indicates a severely diminished pelvic inlet. In this case, if labor was to occur, the fetal head would probably not be able to enter the pelvic outlet. In spite of uterine contractions, the fetal head would not engage, and the presenting part would probably be described as ballotable, or floating. When a measurement such as this is discovered during the prenatal course, the woman is counseled about the need for cesarean birth.

24. Nägele's rule is a method used to determine the estimated date of birth.

25. It is calculated by taking the first day of the LMP, subtracting 3 months, and adding 7 days.

26. Jenny's EDB would be December 29 (± 2 weeks). If you count back February, January, December, it is easy to identify the month. If you set it up as a problem, it is a little more difficult:

March 22 becomes	$3 - 22$
Subtract 3 months	-3
	$0 = 22$
Add 7 days	$+ 7$
EDB	$0 = 29$

   If you remember that January is always the first month, then an answer of "0" becomes December, an answer of "minus 1" would be November, and "minus 2" would be October.

27. Every 4 weeks for first 28 weeks' gestation; every 2 weeks until 36 weeks' gestation; then weekly until childbirth. Note: In some large HMOs this pattern may be somewhat different.

28. Answers may include psychologic status, educational needs, support systems, family functioning, economic status, stability of living conditions.

29. c   30. d   31. e   32. a   33. b

34. You should stress to the woman the importance of contacting her caregiver immediately if she experiences any of the danger signs in pregnancy.

35. urinary frequency, nausea and vomiting, fatigue, breast tenderness, increased vaginal discharge

36. (a) Wear a well-fitting, supportive bra. (b) Dorsiflex the foot to stretch the affected muscle; apply heat. (c) Eat crackers or dry toast before arising in the morning; have small, frequent meals; avoid causative factors; drink carbonated beverages. (d) Increase fluids, dietary fiber, and exercise. (e) Use proper body mechanics; do pelvic-tilt exercise; avoid high-heeled shoes and excessive standing. (f) Void when urge is felt. Increase fluid intake during the day and then decrease fluids only at night to decrease nocturia.

37. b

38. *Actions:* In most clinics and offices, laboratory tests are completed at the initial prenatal visit. Thus you could quickly refer to the results of the hemoglobin and hematocrit to determine if Julie is anemic.

   Analysis: Julie's laboratory values are within normal limits, so you know she is not anemic. It is tempting at this point to simply assume the fatigue is normal because it is so common among pregnant women. However, this assumption might lead you to miss factors in Julie's life that are contributing to the problem, such as extra stress at work, the stress of helping a family member with a sick child, or frequent awakenings at night for trips to the bathroom.

   Actions: An appropriate action might be to provide reassurance while pursuing the matter. You might say, for example, "Many women feel tired during the early months of pregnancy, but sometimes factors or events in the woman's life can add to the fatigue. Is there anything happening in your life that you feel might be contributing to the fatigue?"

   Actions: Julie's indication that her lifestyle is unchanged suggests that the fatigue is a normal part of her pregnancy. At this point you can begin working with her to plan ways for her to get more rest during the day.

39. High-heeled shoes can aggravate back discomfort by increasing the curvature of the spine. They should not be worn if the woman experiences backache or problems with her balance. Theresa may find that she can feel professional but be more comfortable if she switches from high heels to a shoe with a small (1 inch) heel. Shoes should fit properly and feel comfortable.

40. Answers may include the following: exercise regularly, at least three times per week; modify exercise intensity based on symptoms; avoid lying supine to exercise after the first trimester; non-weight-bearing exercises such as swimming and cycling are recommended; wear appropriate clothing and supportive shoes; drink plenty of fluids; stop exercising if warning signs such as dizziness, back pain, palpitations, pubic pain, tachycardia, uterine contractions, or vaginal bleeding develop.

41. The teaching guide on page 385 of your textbook describes one approach. If you are unsure of the methods used in your area, ask your instructor for assistance with this question.

42. Either showers or tub baths are acceptable according to personal preference. Tub baths are contraindicated if there is vaginal bleeding or if the membranes are ruptured because of the risk of introducing infection.

43. Travel by car is fine but can be tiring. Linh should plan to stop about every 2 hours and walk around for about 10 minutes. To avoid bladder trauma, she should void regularly. She should wear both lap and shoulder seat belts. The lap belt should be fastened under her abdomen across her upper thighs.

44. (a) early, (b) delayed until after childbirth if possible

45. Although studies do indicate that light drinkers have a risk of complications similar to that of nondrinkers, there is no known safe level of alcohol consumption during pregnancy and women are best advised to abstain from all alcohol.

46. A possible nursing diagnosis would be **Health-Seeking Behaviors: Information about safe sexual activity during the third trimester related to an expressed desire for further information.** Perhaps you chose **Sexual Dysfunction related to lack of knowledge.** This is a tempting diagnosis because the problem concerns sexual activity, and some people would support this diagnosis. However, because their sexual activity is satisfying to both and they have adapted their practices in light of the pregnancy, they do not meet the definition of a dysfunction. They are simply seeking information.

47. teratogen

48. Answers may include the following: women who delay childbirth tend to be well educated and financially secure; they tend to be emotionally stable; their pregnancies are usually planned, and the baby is wanted; they typically obtain early prenatal care; they are more aware of the realities of having a child.

49. c

50. Answers may include the following: concerns about ability to parent well; about whether they have sufficient energy to care for a baby; about their ability to deal with an older child as they age; about the financial impact of having a college-age child as they near retirement; about the social isolation they feel as older parents.

51. Answers may include the following: peer pressure to engage in sexual activity; needing someone to love; unstable family relationships; competition with mother; desire to punish parent(s); desire for emancipation from home; cultural values that support early pregnancy; unmotivated accident; lack of understanding about contraceptive options; incest; feelings of love for partner.

52. This question gives you a lot of room to plan creatively. Obviously, there is no one right answer. We hope that in planning your clinic you keep in mind that the early adolescent is often quite different in needs and interaction from the late adolescent. Although the older adolescent can often think abstractly, many adolescents are very concrete thinkers and tend to be present oriented and egocentric. Thus it is helpful to use audiovisual aids and provide "hands-on" learning experiences. Activities have more meaning if the adolescent sees them as having a specific value for her.

   In planning, we hope you emphasize a multidisciplinary approach that also includes the father of the child and the parents of the adolescent mother and father (if the adolescents wish them to be involved). This leads to the question of choice: It is important to give these adolescents choices and to help them learn to make appropriate decisions. Thus some guidance may be beneficial; however, too much guidance may keep them from learning how to make choices and decisions.

   Finally, we hope you give some thought to the atmosphere of your clinic: Is it open, nonjudgmental, and supportive? Do the adolescents feel free to ask questions and express fears? Does it feel safe and free of coercion?

53. Iron deficiency anemia, preeclampsia, preterm birth, CPD

54. Ideal weight gain during pregnancy for a woman of normal weight is a gain of 3.5 to 5 lb (1.6 to 2.3 kg) during the first trimester, followed by a gain of about 1 lb (0.4 to 0.5 kg) per week during the second and third trimesters.

55. 300

56. a   57. a   58. i   59. b   60. c

61. g   62. e   63. h   64. d   65. f

66. Pregnant vegetarians often use soybean products such as soybean milk, tofu, and soy protein isolates as a source of protein. Other sources include nuts and lentils. Possible additional sources of calcium include turnip greens, white beans, and almonds.

67. This woman's diet had 4 servings of grain products. This is adequate. She had 4 servings of protein, which is more than adequate. However, because she only had $2^1/_2$ servings of dairy products (recommended is 4) and 3 fruits or vegetables (4 to 6 are recommended), her diet is deficient in these areas.

68. (a) estimated date of birth, (b) estimated date of confinement, (c) estimated date of delivery, (d) fetal activity diary, (e) fetal movement record, (f) gravida, (g) para, (h) recommended dietary allowance

Chapter 8

1. 1; 10

2. exaggerated startle reflex, genitourinary malformations, increased risk of SIDS, IUGR, shorter body length

3. Answers may include the following: general health status, nutritional status, risk of infection, all body systems, woman's knowledge of the impact of substance abuse on her or her fetus.

4. Preferred methods include psychoprophylaxis, regional analgesia or anesthesia such as an epidural or local anesthesia.

5. False. Although there is a tendency to assume that administering an analgesic to a woman who is a substance abuser will increase her addiction, this assumption is not correct. The woman should receive the support necessary to help her deal effectively with the discomfort of labor and birth.

6. Answers include polyuria, polyphagia, polydipsia, weight loss.

7. c   8. d

9. Answers may include changes in insulin requirements; decreased renal threshold for glucose; increased risk of ketoacidosis, insulin shock, and coma; possible acceleration of vascular disease.

10. Answers may include hydramnios, maternal ketoacidosis, fetal death, increased incidence of fetal anomalies, macrosomia, birth trauma, asphyxia.

11. Ms. Cavillo did maintain effective control. Glycosylated hemoglobin is an accurate indicator of a person's long-term control. In the presence of elevated blood glucose levels, hemoglobin A_0 converts to hemoglobin A_{1c} or glycosylated hemoglobin. Because the process is essentially irreversible, elevations indicate that the person has been hyperglycemic. The normal range is approximately 6% to 8%. Thus, Ms. Cavillo's glycohemoglobin level of 7% is within normal limits.

12. Your intervention was very effective. You began by asking Ms. Cavillo for her opinion about ways of helping her keep her appointment. As is often the case, the client herself had obviously thought about the problem and tried to correct it but was unable to do so without assistance. By working in a collaborative way with Ms. Cavillo and the physician, you were able to arrange an effective solution. Good job!

13. Four injections of insulin spread out over the day result in more stable blood sugar levels throughout the day. Moreover, the types of insulin used—generally regular insulin or lispro and NPH—peak at different times.

14. She should exercise after meals when blood sugar levels are high; she should wear diabetic identification and should carry hard candy for a rapid source of sugar. In addition, she should monitor her blood glucose regularly and avoid injecting insulin into an extremity that will soon be used during exercise.

15. a

16. We hope you would tell her that oral hypoglycemics are rarely used during pregnancy because they cross the placenta and have not been well studied. However, one oral medication, glyburide, does not cross the placenta and has been found to be comparable to insulin without evidence of adverse effects in the mother or fetus. This oral agent is now being

used to treat women with gestational diabetes mellitus. (ACOG, 2005).

American College of Obstetricians and Gynecologists (ACOG). (2005). Pregestational diabetes mellitus (ACOG Practice Bulletin No. 60). Washington, DC: Author.

17. Infants who are large at birth generally have mothers who are class A, B, or C diabetics. The infants are exposed to high glucose levels in utero. In response, the fetus produces high levels of insulin and uses the available glucose. This increased use leads to excessive growth (macrosomia).

18. Answers may include maternal serum α-fetoprotein, ultrasound, fetal biophysical profile, nonstress tests, contraction stress test.

19. (a) insufficient hemoglobin production related to nutritional deficiency of iron or folic acid; (b) hemoglobin destruction in an inherited disorder such as sickle cell anemia or thalassemia

20. Iron deficiency

21. See text, pp. 463–464.

22. during labor and birth

23. Answers may include weight loss, fever, oral infections such as thrush, pneumonia, lymph node enlargement, enlarged liver and spleen.

24. Gloves should be worn when contact with blood, body fluids, nonintact skin, or mucous membranes is possible.

25. (a) Asymptomatic. No limitation of physical activity. (b) Slight limitation of physical activity. Asymptomatic at rest; symptoms occur with heavy physical activity. (c) Moderate to marked limitation of physical activity. Symptoms occur during less-than-ordinary physical activity. (d) Inability to carry out any physical activity without discomfort. Even at rest the person experiences symptoms of cardiac insufficiency or anginal pain.

26. Answers may include cough, dyspnea, edema, heart murmurs, palpitations, rales, weight gain.

27. b   28. b

29. Penicillin is started as prophylaxis to prevent recurrent bouts of rheumatic fever and subsequent heart valve damage.

30. Whenever possible, vaginal birth is preferred, using low forceps and a local or regional anesthetic to decrease the stress of the second stage of labor. This procedure also avoids the hazards associated with abdominal surgery for cesarean birth.

31. (a) acquired immunodeficiency syndrome, (b) diabetes mellitus, (c) fetal alcohol syndrome, (d) gestational diabetes mellitus, (e) human immunodeficiency virus, (f) insulin-dependent diabetes mellitus

Chapter 9

1. naturally occurring expulsion of the fetus before viability

2. miscarriage

3. b   4. e   5. d   6. f   7. c   8. a

9. See text, p. 481.

10. A D&C is performed to remove the remainder of the products of conception.

11. Answers may include the following: chromosomal abnormalities, teratogenic drugs, placental abnormalities, faulty implantation, chronic maternal disease, maternal infection, endocrine imbalances.

12. See answer at end of Answer Key on pp. 242–243.

13. Answers may include the following: cervical trauma, congenital cervical structural defects, uterine anomalies.

14. Shirodkar-Barter operation (cerclage)

15. Implantation of the blastocyst in a site other than the endometrial lining of the uterus

16. fallopian tubes

17. See text, pp. 484–485.

18. d   19. a

20. Continued high or rising hCG levels are abnormal and may indicate the development of choriocarcinoma. Periodic examinations are necessary to detect rising levels. Ms. Chan should avoid pregnancy because otherwise it would be difficult to tell whether elevated hCG levels were related to pregnancy or developing malignancy.

21. Excessive vomiting during pregnancy

22. (a) control vomiting, (b) correct dehydration, (c) restore electrolyte balance, (d) maintain adequate nutrition

23. Rupture of the membranes before 37 weeks' gestation

24. respiratory distress syndrome (RDS)

25. infection

26. Nitrazine paper; blue or blue-green; alkaline

27. Answers may include the following: continue bed rest with bathroom privileges; monitor temperature four times daily; avoid sexual intercourse, douches, and tampons; contact

physician if she has fever, uterine tenderness, contractions, increased leakage of fluid, decreased fetal movement, foul-smelling vaginal discharge.

28. previous preterm birth, smoking 15 cigarettes a day, history of pyelonephritis, bleeding at 14 weeks' gestation, low socioeconomic level

29. To answer Ms. Benitah, you need to include the following: She will need to watch for signs of preterm labor, which include uterine contractions every 10 minutes or less, mild menstrual-like cramps felt low in the abdomen, feelings of pelvic pressure, low backache that is constant or comes and goes, a change in vaginal discharge, and abdominal cramping with or without diarrhea.

    Teach her to lie down on her side or tilted to one side with a pillow. She may then place her fingertips on the fundus of the uterus. She checks for contractions (hardening or tightening) for about 1 hour. If contractions are felt every 10 minutes for 1 hour, she needs to call her healthcare provider.

30. A contraction will feel like a hardening or tightening of the uterus. She may also note a backache that comes and goes on a regular pattern of every 10 minutes. This may be associated with contractions.

31. Y   32. Y   33. N   34. N

35. N   36. Y   37. Y   38. N

39. Magnesium sulfate decreases the frequency and intensity of uterine contractions.

40. (a) 4 to 6, (b) 1 to 4

41. calcium

42. See text, pp. 499–500.

43. Helen Polawski exhibits a number of factors that contraindicate beginning therapy to stop her labor. She is 5 cm dilated, and her contractions indicate active labor. Her membranes have been ruptured for just short of 24 hours, and although you do not know the cause of her low-grade fever, you should suspect amnionitis at this point. These factors would lead you to answer "no." The most pressing nursing goal is probably to prepare her for childbirth. With three previous births, a small baby this time (34 weeks' gestation), and 5 cm dilatation with active labor, the birth may be just a few minutes away.

44. (a) 3, (b) 4, (c) NA, (d) 2, (e) 1, (f) NA, (g) NA

45. *Actions:* We hope you would check Ms. Sherbo's blood pressure and test her urine for protein.

    Analysis: Ms. Sherbo's BP is elevated significantly. An increase of 30/15 indicates mild preeclampsia. Ms. Sherbo's BP has increased 42/26, her urine contains protein, and she has had a major weight gain. Her symptoms indicate more than mild preeclampsia. We hope that at this point you would assess Rita for further signs of severe preeclampsia.

    Assessments: At this point you could ask Ms. Sherbo about additional symptoms such as headache, visual changes, or epigastric pain. You can quickly assess deep tendon reflexes and observe for evidence of edema.

    Actions: You now have a clear picture of Ms. Sherbo's status and should report your findings to the physician. Your preliminary assessments will help the physician realize the need to see Ms. Sherbo quickly. Because you would expect the physician to admit Ms. Sherbo to the hospital, you can quickly confirm his or her intentions and begin the necessary procedures for admission. You will thus avoid unnecessary delays for Ms. Sherbo.

    Analysis: You know that the unexpected hospitalization must be stressful for Ms. Sherbo. You also realize that she must have many questions and concerns.

    Actions: Take the time to explain things to Ms. Sherbo and answer her questions. She will probably be worried about the impact of the preeclampsia on her unborn child and may also be worried about the problems caused for her family by her hospitalization. Having an opportunity to talk, plan, and consider her alternatives will be especially helpful. You can also offer to contact Ms. Sherbo's family and explain the situation. If she is upset, it may be necessary to arrange with them to transport her to the hospital. Any support and assistance you can provide will be very helpful to her.

46. See text, pp. 507–508.

47. Grand mal seizures or coma

48. c

49. See text, pp. 509–510.

50. d

51. (a) 6, (b) 20, (c) 2

52. Answers include diminished or absent reflexes, depressed respirations, marked lethargy.

53. hemolysis, elevated liver enzymes, low platelet count

54. 3 + DTRs are brisker than average but may not be abnormal.

55. To assess for clonus, quickly dorsiflex the woman's foot. When there is hyperreflexia, the

foot will jerk. Each movement (jerk) is counted, so two beats of clonus means there were two movements after the foot was dorsiflexed.

56. If you answered "no," you were right on target. Carolyn Lorenzo is not a candidate for RhoGAM because her indirect Coombs' test indicates that she has already been sensitized to Rh+ blood and has developed antibodies. Since her first baby was Rh−, it is not known when Carolyn became sensitized. She may have had an undiagnosed pregnancy that ended in early miscarriage, she may have had a blood transfusion with Rh+ blood, or she may have had a small placental bleed during this pregnancy. Regardless of when it occurred, she needs a clear explanation of the risks she faces for hemolytic disease in subsequent pregnancies and her newborn needs to be evaluated carefully.

57. It provides passive antibody protection against Rh antigens.

58. See text, pp. 527–528.

59. a   60. b

61. first

62. d   63. a   64. c   65. b

66. We hope you would tell her that, although there is a lower incidence of herpes infection in infants born by cesarean, cesarean birth is not guaranteed to prevent herpes infection in the newborn. Moreover, it does carry the risk of surgery for the mother. Currently, the recommended approach to deciding about the route of birth is to examine the woman carefully for signs of lesions and ask her about the presence of any prodromal symptoms. If either is present, cesarean birth is indicated. If no signs of infection are present, she will probably give birth vaginally. Ms. Grebliunas may also find it helpful to talk with her caregiver about taking an oral antiviral medication such as acyclovir (Zovirax), beginning several weeks before her anticipated due date in order to suppress the infection.

67. a

68. (a) cytomegalic inclusion disease; (b) cytomegalovirus; (c) disseminated intravascular coagulation; (d) deep tendon reflexes; (e) sexually transmitted disease; (f) sexually transmitted infection.

Interventions	Rationale	Expected Outcome
Goals: Client/husband will: begin the process of anticipatory grieving AEB: Expressions of feelings of loss, spiritual beliefs about the loss of the child, signs of coping such as the ability to make mutual decisions		
Assessments:		
• Assess past experiences of client/husband with loss.	People who have experienced prior losses and have coped successfully have some understanding of the	Woman and her husband express their thoughts and feelings about the loss.
• Assess existing support systems and current grief work.	grieving process and have a starting point for coping. People who have not experienced any major loss may need more information about the grief process, normal responses, and the length of time it takes.	Woman and her husband identify plans to use available social support.
Nursing Interventions:		
• Encourage expression of feelings about the loss.	The ability to verbalize feelings about the loss is a healthy first step in the grieving process.	
• Include husband and significant others in discussion as appropriate.		
• Discuss differences in individual patterns of grieving (i.e., male vs. female).	The knowledge that men and women often deal with loss differently may help couples avoid misinterpreting a partner's responses (or apparent lack of response) to a situation.	

(continued)

Interventions	Rationale	Expected Outcome
• Encourage woman and her husband to implement cultural, religious, and social customs associated with the loss. Collaborative: • With the couple's approval, arrange for a chaplain or spiritual leader to visit and assist with planning if appropriate.	Cultural practices help families deal with loss and provide opportunities for the community to support the grieving couple.	

12. Based on the case scenario, the most pertinent responses could include:

    Collaborative problems: 1. Hemorrhage

                                          2. Infection

    Nursing diagnosis: Grieving, anticipatory
    Defining characteristics:
    Crying, Althea's expressions of guilt that she may have done something "wrong," husband's expression of sorrow and loss.

Chapter 10

1. Ultrasound can be used for all of the indications; however, assistance and guidance with an amniocentesis takes place in the second trimester.

2. Some advantages of ultrasound testing include the following: transabdominal method is noninvasive, it is a generally painless procedure with the exception of discomfort from a full bladder (for ultrasound in the first two trimesters), there is no radiation involved, it allows for differentiation of soft tissues, immediate information may be gained.

3. Early pregnancy uses include determination of gestational sac and placement of the sac, identification of the embryo or fetus, number of embryos or fetuses, presence or absence of fetal heart activity, fetal measurements for growth, location of the placenta. Late pregnancy uses include following fetal growth patterns, location of placenta, validating fetal presentation and position, investigating congenital anomalies or problems, assessing amount of amniotic fluid, completion of biophysical profile, location of umbilical cord for cordocentesis.

4. To date, there are no known ill effects from ultrasound. Ultrasound has been in use for more than 30 years.

5. At this time, Sherry's uterus is lower than expected and she should have felt fetal movement. Ultrasound can provide information regarding the gestation.

6. Explain that she will have to drink water to fill her bladder; then an abdominal or vaginal ultrasound probe will be used. The test should not be uncomfortable.

7. a

8. (a) Your teaching plan should include points such as begin assessing at about 30 to 32 weeks; during rest periods, gently place her hand on the fundus to detect fetal movement and to feel uterine contractions. See text for further information. (b) Her attentiveness during each assessment period will be important. The fetus tends to move more after the mother has eaten. It is important that the mother understand the fetus has periods of sleep, during which fetal movement may not be felt for 20 to 40 minutes.

9. To determine fetal well-being, measured by the ability of the fetus to respond to its body movement with an acceleration of the FHR.

10. See text, pp. 552–555.

11. See text, pp. 552–555.

12. Reactive NST. This test demonstrates that the fetus is able to respond to movement with an acceleration of the FHR. The fetus is not stressed and has reserve to cope with changes in the environment.

13. Figure 10–1, *A* is reactive. Figure 10–1, *B* is nonreactive.

14. A vibroacoustic stimulation (VAS) test may be used when the NST is nonreactive. A sound is transmitted through the maternal abdomen into the uterus. A fetus who is asleep will respond to the sound with an acceleration in FHR. If the fetus is stressed and unable to respond, the NST will remain nonreactive and further assessment is needed immediately.

15. (a) The five biophysical variables are fetal breathing movements, gross body movements,

fetal tone, reactive fetal heart rate, qualitative amniotic fluid volume. (b) Each biophysical variable is scored as 2 or A "good" score is 10 (2 points on each variable) or 8 (as long as amniotic fluid volume received a score of 2). (c) In any situation in which the fetus is thought to be at risk due to maternal or fetal factors. (d) Decreased amniotic fluid is associated with oligohydramnios. The fetus is at increased risk because the umbilical cord does not have enough fluid to float in and may become compressed. (e) Your teaching plan should include what the test is; the anticipated usefulness, benefits, risks, and interpretations of the results; and whom to contact for further information.

16. Maternal indications for a CST include diabetes mellitus and suspected postmaturity. Fetal indications include IUGR, reactive NST, and abnormal or suspicious BPP.

17. Contraindications include third trimester bleeding, previous cesarean birth with classic uterine incision, presence of placenta previa.

18. See text, pp. 556–560.

19. A BSST involves stimulating endogenous oxytocin. A CST depends on IV administration of oxytocin (exogenous).

20. a   21. b

22. (a) The CST tracing is negative. (b) There are no late decelerations with uterine contractions. Note three contractions have occurred in just over 8 minutes.

23. Draw any of the test results. Visualization of results helps you learn.

24. MSAFP is a *screening* test that uses maternal hormone levels to determine if a mother is *at risk* for certain abnormalities such as neural tube defects, Down syndrome, and trisomy 18. The test cannot screen for structural or other types of birth defects.

25. The CVS is a test that can be done as early as 9 weeks (and up to 12 weeks) to detect genetic, metabolic, and DNA abnormalities in the developing fetus. A CVS is performed by obtaining a sample of chorionic villi from the edge of the developing placenta. An amniocentesis involves withdrawing amniotic fluid from the uterine cavity and can test for genetic, metabolic, and DNA abnormalities. The amniocentesis can also screen for neural tube defects. The CVS has twice the risk of spontaneous abortion and also carries a risk of limb-reduction abnormalities.

26. Amniocentesis provides a specimen of amniotic fluid for testing.

27. Ultrasound guidance is essential.

28. Nursing interventions during an amniocentesis should include the following: prepare the equipment, cleanse the abdomen, assess the maternal vital signs and the FHR before amniocentesis and after the procedure is completed, document amniocentesis in the client's chart, provide information and support to the client.

29. Complications may include infection (from contamination of the uterine contents with pathogens), continued leakage of amniotic fluid (from failure of the puncture site to close), bleeding (from puncture of the placenta or umbilical cord), irritation of the uterus that results in contractions (is treated with a beta-sympathomimetic).

30. The L/S ratio test determines the amount of lecithin to sphingomyelin. Normal results are 2:1 and indicate that the fetus has sufficient surfactant to support extrauterine respirations. The phosphatidylglycerol test determines the presence or absence of another key phospholipid in surfactant. The presence of phosphatidylglycerol also indicates that adequate amounts of stable surfactant are present.

31. *Actions:* You need to know more about the contraction characteristics (such as frequency, duration, and intensity of contractions) and whether there are any additional signs of labor. *Actions:* You will need to reiterate the discharge instructions, which should include signs of labor, how to assess uterine contractions, and signs of infections.

32. The correct answer is yes. The L/S ratio is mature, and the presence of PG is also associated with fetal lung maturity.

33. (a) amniotic fluid index, (b) breast self-stimulation test, (c) biophysical profile, (d) crown–rump length, (e) contraction stress test, (f) chorionic villi sampling, (g) fetal heart rate, (h) femur length, (i) head circumference, (j) intrauterine growth restriction, (k) lecithin-sphingomyelin ratio, (l) maternal serum alpha-fetoprotein, (m) nonstress test, (n) phosphatidylglycerol, (o) ultrasound, (p) vibroacoustic stimulation, (q) nuchal translucency test.

Chapter 11

1. (a) The size and shape of the maternal pelvis determine whether a fetus (of average birth weight) can pass through and be born. For

example, if the expectant woman's pelvic inlet has a very small transverse, the fetal head may be blocked from entering the birth passage. Uterine contractions may occur, but the fetal head cannot enter the inlet.

A vaginal examination would reveal a cervix that is very difficult to reach (cervix would probably be high up in the vaginal canal), and if the fetal head can be reached, it would move away (upward) from the examiner's gloved finger (because the fetal head is not *engaged*).

In this example, the nurse, certified nurse-midwife, or physician must first determine if "true" labor exists and, second, if this fetal head is able to enter this pelvic inlet. The described example is only one of the possible implications.

(b) Psychosocial considerations of labor and birth continue to be explored through qualitative research methods. What the expectant woman brings to the labor and birth may have an enormous effect on the labor process. Is the woman confident that she can make it through the birth journey? Will she be able to handle the pain? Does she have support (partner and labor nurse)?

2. The inlet and pelvic cavity of the adult gynecoid pelvis are rounded; therefore, all the pelvic diameters are more likely to be adequate for the fetus to pass through during labor and birth. The anthropoid pelvis tends to be more heart shaped but still provides adequate measurements for the fetus to pass through.

3. The android (typical male) pelvis is wide from front to back but very narrow from side to side. This interferes with descent of the fetus into the inlet. The platypelloid pelvic inlet is very wide from side to side, so descent of the fetal head into the pelvis is more likely than with an android; however, the inlet is very narrow front to back and this interferes with internal rotation.

4. See text, p. 578.

5. b   6. c

7. (a) occipital bone, (b) lambdoidal suture, (c) posterior fontanelle, (d) sagittal suture, (e) parietal bone, (f) coronal suture, (g) anterior fontanelle, (h) mitotic suture

8. The sutures of the fetal skull are membranous spaces between the cranial bones. The intersections of the sutures are called fontanelles.

9. b   10. c   11. d   12. a

13. The anterior and posterior fontanelles are the intersections between the sutures. The anterior fontanelle allows growth of the brain by

remaining unossified for as long as 18 months. The posterior fontanelle closes between 8 and 12 weeks after birth. During labor and birth, the descent and position of the fetal head can be assessed by palpating the posterior suture.

14. (a) The anterior fontanelle is located between the coronal, frontal, and sagittal suture and is diamond shaped. (b) The posterior fontanelle is located between the sagittal and the lambdoidal suture and is triangular in shape.

15. (a) anterior fontanelle, (b) vertex, (c) posterior fontanelle, (d) occiput, (e) mastoid fontanelle, (f) mentum (chin), (g) sphenoid fontanelle, (h) sinciput (brow)

16. *View A.* (a) suboccipitobregmatic, (b) 9.5 cm, (c) occipitofrontal, (d) 11.75 cm, (e) occipitomental, (f) 13.5 cm.

View B. (g) biparietal diameter, (h) 9.25 cm, (i) bitemporal diameter, (j) 8 cm

17. b   18. c   19. a

20. See text, p. 579.

21. The fetal presentation is determined by fetal lie and by the body part of the fetus that enters the mother's pelvis first.

22. Vertex, military, brow, face

23. Complete breech (fetal buttocks down against cervix), frank breech (fetal buttocks down against cervix, fetal legs up against abdomen and chest), footling (one or both feet are against the cervix).

24. (a) cephalic presentation, (b) ROA, (c) presenting part—occiput

25. (a) cephalic presentation, (b) LOP, (c) presenting part—occiput

26. (a) cephalic presentation, (b) LOA, (c) presenting part—occiput

27. (a) cephalic presentation, (b) LOT, (c) presenting part—occiput

28. (a) cephalic presentation, (b) ROP, (c) presenting part—occiput

29. (a) breech presentation, (b) LSA, (c) presenting part—sacrum

30. (a) breech presentation, (b) RSA, (c) presenting part—sacrum

31. (a) cephalic (face) presentation, (b) LMA, (c) presenting part—mentum

32. (a) cephalic (face) presentation, (b) RMP, (c) presenting part—mentum

33. (a) breech presentation, (b) LSP, (c) presenting part—sacrum

34. (a) transverse lie, (b) LAPA, (c) presenting part—shoulder

35. (a) cephalic (face) presentation, (b) RMA,
    (c) presenting part—mentum

36. (a) breech presentation, (b) single footling,
    (c) presenting part—single footling

    If you had difficulty with this question, refer
    back to the definitions of presentation and position.
    It may also help to use a model of a pelvis with a
    fetus. This is an important aspect, so keep at it.

37. Methods include Leopold's maneuvers, visual
    inspection of the maternal abdomen, location of
    fetal heart rate, vaginal examination, assessment
    of the mother's greatest area of discomfort
    (posterior position is associated with severe
    backache), visualization by ultrasound.

38. Engagement of the presenting part occurs when
    the largest diameter of the presenting part
    reaches or passes through the pelvic inlet.

39. None. Engagement provides information about
    the inlet but not about the midpelvis or outlet.
    Fetal descent would provide information about
    the midpelvis and outlet.

40. Leopold's maneuvers and vaginal examinations
    can be used to determine engagement.

41. Questions such as the following should be
    directed toward changes the mother might feel
    once engagement has occurred. (a) "Have you
    recently noticed a change in the way your clothes
    fit?" Rationale: As the fetal head drops into the
    inlet, there may be a change in the shape of the
    abdomen. It may seem that the baby has dropped
    down and away from the mother's body. This
    causes a change in the way her clothes fit.
    (b) "Have you recently noticed that you have to
    urinate more frequently?" Rationale: As the fetus
    descends into the pelvis, there may be more
    pressure on the bladder. (c) "Have you noticed
    more discomfort in your pelvic area and your
    thighs?" Rationale: As the fetus descends into the
    pelvis, there may be more discomfort. There may
    also be increased pressure from vasocongestion
    of the areas below the pelvis (that is, the perineum
    and the lower extremities). (d) "Have you noticed
    easier breathing?" Rationale: As the fetus
    descends into the pelvis, there may be less
    pressure on the diaphragm.

    Any of these changes may suggest that
    engagement has occurred, but they are not
    diagnostic.

42. *Station* refers to the relationship of the presenting
    part to an imaginary line drawn between the
    ischial spines of the maternal pelvis.

43. Minus (−) 1 station means the presenting part is
    1 cm above the ischial spines.

44. Failure to descend may be associated with
    cephalopelvic disproportion, malposition,
    malpresentation, asynclitism, or multiple
    pregnancy.

45. c   46. b   47. e   48. d   49. a   50. f

51. (a) increment, (b) acme, (c) decrement,
    (d) duration, (e) frequency

52. Factors may include Amy's desire for this baby,
    amount of education (general and childbirth),
    coping skills, support from others, worry about
    the pregnancy or about being a parent, view of
    self, role changes, worry about finances, fear
    that she will not be able to tolerate the labor
    and birth in the way she wishes, and association
    of pregnancy, labor, and/or birth with previous
    abuse.

53. Culture shapes our worldview and our ideas
    about role, behavior, customs, the way we
    respond to challenges or pain, what we want
    for comfort, eating and drinking preferences,
    and so on.

54. c   55. c   56. d

57. *First:* from beginning of true labor to complete
    dilatation. *Second:* from complete dilatation to
    birth of baby. *Third:* from birth of baby to birth
    of placenta. *Fourth:* from birth of placenta to
    2 to 4 hours after birth.

58. (a) Latent, (b) active, (c) transitional

59. First stage, latent phase

60. (a) 1.2 cm/hr, (b) 1.5 cm/hr for a multigravida

61. Frequency every 2 to 2.5 minutes, duration 60 to
    75 seconds, intensity strong.

62. Physiologic causes of pain during labor include
    the following: uterine muscle hypoxia as
    contractions occur and become longer, closer,
    and stronger; stretching of the cervix as it dilates
    and effaces; pressure of the presenting part on
    the cervix; stretching of the vaginal and perineal
    tissues; exhaustion.

63. Key factors include psychosocial, cultural factors
    such as age, maturity level, educational level,
    amount of knowledge regarding childbirth,
    availability of supportive person, coping abilities,
    ability to make decisions and make wishes
    known, cultural expectations, and opportunities
    for expressions of pain, fear, and anxiety.

64. (a) Left-acromion-dorsal-anterior, (b) left-
    acromion-dorsal-posterior, (c) left-mentum-
    anterior, (d) left-mentum-posterior, and last
    menstrual period, (e) left-mentum-transverse,
    (f) left-occiput-anterior, (g) left-occiput-
    posterior, (h) left-occiput-transverse,
    (i) left-sacrum-anterior, (j) left-sacrum-posterior,

(k) left-sacrum-transverse, (l) right-mentum-anterior, (m) right-mentum-posterior, (n) right-mentum-transverse, (o) right-occiput-anterior, (p) rupture of membranes, (q) right-occiput-posterior, (r) right-occiput-transverse, (s) right-sacrum-anterior, (t) right-sacrum-posterior, (u) right-sacrum-transverse, (v) spontaneous rupture of membranes, (w) artificial rupture of membranes

Chapter 12

1. The answers will depend on the role your friend takes. Answer all the questions you can. Practice different ways of phrasing questions so that you are best able to elicit answers to the questions.

2. There are four pertinent assessments of uterine contractions: intensity, frequency, duration, and the client's response to the contractions.

3. Fingertips are more sensitive and provide less pressure.

4. Contraction frequency 10 to 20 minutes, duration 15 to 20 seconds, mild intensity; progressing to frequency 5 to 7 minutes, duration 30 to 40 seconds, moderate intensity.

5. (a) Every 5 minutes, (b) 30 seconds, (c) mild

6.
Contraction Begins	*Contraction Ends*
0500:00	0500:40
	(duration 40 seconds)
0505:00	0505:40
(frequency 5 min)	(duration 40 seconds)
0508:00	0508:45
(frequency 3 min)	(duration 45 seconds)
0511:00	0511:45
(frequency 3 min)	(duration 45 seconds)

   Remember, frequency is the time from the beginning of one contraction to the beginning of the next contraction. (a) The frequency indicated by the first two contractions is 5 minutes; the frequency from the second through the fourth contraction is 3 minutes. This would be recorded as every 3 to 5 minutes. (b) The duration is 40 to 45 seconds.

7. Mild feels like a slightly contracted biceps muscle. Moderate is similar to a tightly contracted biceps muscle. Strong is similar to feeling the back of your hand: it cannot be indented by your fingers.

8. (a) Locate the FHR by beginning in the lower left segment of the maternal uterus and then work in ever-enlarging circles until the FHR is heard. (b) You check the maternal pulse and listen to the FHR to make sure that the rates are different. The FHR should be more rapid than that of the normal laboring woman. (c) It is best to listen for at least 30 seconds, and every so often you should listen for 60 seconds. During the labor, it is important to listen through a contraction to detect any slowing of the heart rate if an electronic fetal monitor is not being used. Guidelines for when to listen in low-risk situations are as follows: every 30 minutes during the first stage (active and transition phase), every 15 minutes during the second stage. It is important to listen to FHR immediately after the rupture of amniotic membranes, if the amniotic fluid has a greenish color (meconium staining), after an enema if given, after any analgesic or regional block, and with any significant change of maternal vital signs or change in fetal activity.

9. The woman should be lying on her back with a small pillow under her head. The knees are drawn up, with feet flat on the bed to increase relaxation of the abdominal muscles.

10. (a) cephalic, (b) right occiput. Note that you were not given enough specific information to determine whether the right (R) occiput (O) was anterior (ROA) or posterior (ROP). Think through what your hands would feel if the fetus was LOA, LOP, or RSA (right-sacrum-anterior).

11. The membrane status is ascertained beforehand because the lubricant used for the vaginal examination can change the reactivity of the Nitrazine test tape and thereby give a false reading.

12. Intact membranes act as a dilating wedge against the cervix and protect the fetal head from compression against the cervix.

13. Ruptured of membranes (ROM) allow for greater pressure to be applied to the cervix during contractions by the fetal head and therefore may hasten cervical dilatation and effacement. Once membranes are ruptured, there is an open pathway into the uterus and infection may occur in the uterine cavity if ROM is prolonged.

14. Most sources recommend that the birth occur within 24 hours after rupture of membranes because after that time the incidence of infection increases. You will need to know when they rupture to be able to keep track of the 24 hours.

15. When membranes rupture, the umbilical cord may prolapse (umbilical cord may be washed down ahead of the fetal head into the cervix or vagina). This will most likely be indicated by a decrease in the FHR.

16. To assist Ann, consider the following: you need to assess her information base and understanding of the benefits and risks of amniotomy. Provide additional information as needed. Make sure she understands the risks and benefits and has an opportunity to talk further with her certified nurse-midwife or physician.

17. Your response might be something like: "Mrs. X would prefer not to have an amniotomy done."

18. You might say, "Mrs. X has said she would prefer not to have an amniotomy. Is there something you are finding that she needs to know to reconsider her decision?" You are in a position to continue to be the client advocate. As you ask further questions, be direct and work to facilitate the exchange of information between Mrs. X and her physician.

19. (a) The membranes are intact. The Nitrazine test is negative. (b) The most likely source of the clear fluid is the bladder.

20. (a) A number of assessments are made while performing a vaginal examination. You can determine cervical effacement and dilatation; determine fetal descent, station, position, and presentation; and assess pelvic measurements. (b) Position her in low-Fowler's with her heels together and knees out to the side. Use the sheet or a warm blanket to drape her legs and vulva. Make sure the door to the room is closed and the curtains around the bed are closed.

21. (a) Factors leading to anxiety could include fear of pain, emotional stress, underlying psychologic disorders, or a history of incest, rape, or sexual assault. (b) Provide Ann with a thorough explanation of why the exam is needed and what information will be obtained. Encourage her to relax with slow breathing in through her nose and out through her mouth. Stay with her throughout the exam and encourage her to keep her abdomen and buttocks relaxed. Allow her support person to remain with her throughout the exam if she prefers.

22. (a) 3 cm. If you did not answer this correctly, refer to appendix on cervical dilatations in your textbook. (b) Cephalic. The head feels firm compared to the softer tissues of its buttocks when the fetus is in a breech presentation. (c) Left occiput anterior (LOA). The triangular shape is the posterior fontanelle. If it is felt in the upper portion of the cervix, the fetus is LOA. Refer to Figure 23–3 (or your textbook) for help in visualizing this fetal position. (d) Rupture of capillaries in the cervix.

23. Aspects of the Lamaze breathing are presented in Chapter 24.

24. You can provide Roy with information and opportunities for questions. He can support Ann with comfort measures such as fluids, a comfortable place to sit, and encouragement.

25. Fetal baseline refers to the average FHR obtained during a 10-minute period of monitoring. Fetal tachycardia is a sustained rate of 160 beats per minute or above. Fetal bradycardia is a rate less than 110 beats per minute. Baseline variability should be present. Deceleration is the periodic decrease in FHR from the normal baseline. For definitions of early, late, and variable deceleration, see answer to question 32.

26. (a) Electronic fetal monitor, (b) fetal heart rate, (c) uterine activity

27. (a) 110, (b) 160, (c) present, (d) no

28. The possible causes of fetal tachycardia include prematurity, mild or chronic fetal hypoxia, fetal infection, frequent repetitive fetal movements, maternal anxiety, maternal drugs, high maternal temperature, and fetal arrhythmias.

29. The possible causes of fetal bradycardia include fetal hypoxia; sudden hypoxemia; arrhythmia, such as congenital heart block; hypothermia; and drugs, such as beta-adrenergic blocking agents (anesthetic agent used for paracervical block).

30. Turn the mother onto her other side and continue to reposition as needed. Increase intravenous fluid rate. If she is receiving Pitocin, discontinue the infusion. Apply oxygen via face mask. Perform a vaginal examination to rule out a cord prolapse and assess cervical change. Provide scalp stimulation in an attempt to raise the FHR. Notify the attending physician or CNM. If heart rate does not recover, anticipate and have other nurses assist with preparations for emergency cesarean birth.

31. The possible causes of changes in baseline variability include maternal medications, fetal rest, gestation of less than 32 weeks, fetal hypoxia and acidosis, and fetal malformation.

32. (a) Early deceleration occurs when the fetal head is compressed and cerebral blood flow is decreased, which leads to central vagal stimulation and results in a slowing of the FHR. (b) Late deceleration is caused by uteroplacental insufficiency resulting from decreased blood flow and oxygen transfer to the fetus through the intervillous spaces during uterine contractions. (c) Variable deceleration occurs if the umbilical cord becomes compressed.

33. (a) every 1.5 to 2 minutes, (b) 40 to 60 seconds. Early decelerations.

34. Contraction frequency: 1 minute to 1 minute 40 seconds; duration: 40 to 80 seconds. Type of FHR pattern: late decelerations. Variability: Average. Contraction frequency is NOT within normal expectations. Contractions should not exceed a frequency of every 2 minutes or a duration of more than 75 (or at most 90) seconds.

35. Contraction frequency: Every 2 minutes; duration: 50 to 60 seconds. Type of FHR pattern: Variable decelerations.

36. Late decelerations: Because late decelerations are caused by uteroplacental insufficiency, all nursing actions should be directed toward increasing perfusion to the placenta and fetus. Interventions would include turning the laboring woman to her side (left or right); checking maternal BP for hypotension and either increasing IV flow rate (with physiologic fluid) or beginning an IV if hypotension is present; starting oxygen per face mask; and of course, immediately reassessing for expected improvement as a result of the interventions and notifying the certified nurse-midwife or physician. Variable decelerations are caused by compression on the fetal umbilical cord. Nursing actions would be focused on relieving the cord compression by changing the woman's position.

37. (a) The client history should indicate no use of narcotics because Stadol will precipitate a withdrawal. Maternal knowledge base regarding the medication, maternal BP, and FHR status should be assessed before admission of the medication. (b) Assess maternal BP, respirations, pulse, and FHR status. (c) Laboring woman is able to rest between contractions and has increased comfort.

38. Transition phase of the first stage of labor.

39. (a) Nursing interventions may include the following: Stand close by with your face near to hers and talk to her very quietly in a supportive voice (e.g., "I will stay with you, breathe with me, watch me, take a breath, your contraction is ending, take a cleansing breath and rest"); do not touch her (in transition, women do not usually like to be touched); keep the environment quiet to decrease stimulation; provide support and encouragement to both partners; demonstrate confidence in your abilities to assist the couple; do not leave her alone; be accepting and nonjudgmental of her coping skills, but do not allow her to hurt another person (e.g., biting her support person). All of these nursing interventions are aimed at increasing support, comfort, trust, and rapport, and providing a caring and supportive environment. (b) Woman is able to rest between contractions, is exhibiting less panicky behavior, is able to breathe with contractions, appears to have increased comfort, is less restless, face and body relaxes.

40. (a) Hyperventilation (breathing too fast and deeply with contractions). (b) Talk with her and encourage her to slow her respirations; breathe with her; have her cup her hands in around her mouth and breathe in and out in her hands during contractions, and breathe into a paper bag. You must remember that the woman is experiencing an acute sense that she must breathe faster and deeper and it is difficult for her to believe that she needs to change that pattern. Stay with her and provide encouragement and support until the pattern improves. (c) See Table 24–7, p. 662.

41. (a) 10, (b) second stage

42. Signs include uncontrollable urge to bear down, increased bloody show, bulging of the perineum, and crowning of the fetal head.

43. See text, pp. 665–667; and Table 24–9, p. 665.

44. See text, pp. 661–664.

45. Provide continuous encouragement for resting between contractions, provide support during pushing efforts, keep couple informed of progress, and provide comfort measures (cool cloth over forehead, ice chips, privacy, assistance with positioning, and support of body parts).

46. Indications include a short perineum that appears that it will tear during birth, and the need to enlarge the vaginal opening for the use of forceps or a vacuum extractor to hasten the second stage.

47. See Figure 27–3.

48. See text, pp. 774–777.

49. *Prenatal:* Exercise, tailor sitting, massage the perineum with oil.

    Labor and birth: Allow the mother to respond to the natural urge to push instead of encouraging her to push before she feels a strong urge (work with her body, not the desires of attending nurses and physician or certified nurse-midwife). During pushing, stretch the perineum slightly by massaging gently with gloved fingers and warmed solution. Encourage woman to respond to what her body is directing her to do, and to push as much as she feels comfortable doing. Encourage gentle pushing when the fetal head is born.

50. To prevent the fetal head from emerging rapidly and tearing the vaginal tissues.

51. To remove secretions that have filled the fetal mouth, nose, and throat.

52. (a) Circle assessments in Figure 12–5. (b) The Apgar score is 8. One point off for respiratory effort and one point off for color. (c) Apgar scores are assessed at 1 and 5 minutes past birth.

53. A pink body indicates that the baby's heartbeat and respirations are in the normal range and the baby is probably not having difficulty. You could probably assume that the heart rate would be scored 2, and the respiratory effort would also meet the criteria for a score of 2. As long as the baby has not received any narcotics or medications that cause muscle relaxation, you could also assume that the baby will have a 2 on muscle tone and reflex irritability.

    Overall, the heart rate and then respiration are the most important factors, because without them the other characteristics are not possible. Think about it: you cannot have a pink body and depressed or no respirations, and you certainly cannot have an absence of heartbeat.

54. Dry newborn with warmed blankets, place newborn skin to skin on mother's chest, place under radiant heater.

55. To prevent evaporative heat loss.

56. The radiant heater works by warming the surface that the heat touches; therefore, the newborn should be unclothed so the skin is warmed.

57. (a) The umbilical vessels and the kidneys are formed embryonically at about the same time. The absence of one artery may indicate kidney problems. (b) Two arteries and one vein should be present.

58. Answers include the following: application of name bands, footprinting.

59. Head slightly down with head to the side.

60. Stimulation of the vagus nerve in the back of the throat with subsequent bradycardia.

61. The brief physical assessment of the newborn should include overall size and general appearance, posture and movements, rate and irregularities of the apical pulse, and respirations (rate, presence of retractions, grunting).

    If the newborn is stable, you may continue by assessing the head (general appearance, discoloration, fontanelles, flaring of nostrils, condition of palate), the neck (webbing or any limitation of movement), the abdomen (size, shape, contour, abnormal pulsations, number of vessels in umbilical cord), extremities (asymmetry, movement, number of digits), skin (discolorations, edema), and elimination (record on newborn record any voiding or stools).

62. Place newborn baby skin to skin on mother's chest, encourage the mother and father to touch their baby, provide support in interacting with the baby (the environment in the birthing/ delivery room may suggest that the parents need to "not touch"), and point out similarities of the baby to the parents.

63. Talking to the baby; stroking, patting, and holding the baby; talking in a higher voice; looking for similarities with family members; calling the baby by name; snuggling; *en face* position; looking for eye contact.

64. Further protrusion of the umbilical cord out of the vagina, a gush of vaginal bleeding, a change in the shape of the uterus, a rise of the fundus in the abdomen.

65. (a) Schultze expulsion results in the center of the placenta separating from the endometrial wall; the rest of the placenta is therefore pulled off. The Duncan separation begins with a margin of the center separating; then the rest of the placenta is pulled off. (b) A Schultze placenta appears with the fetal side (shiny). With a Duncan separation, the maternal side (more rough and ragged looking because it is the cotyledons) shows.

66. Normal placentas detach anywhere from immediately after the birth of the baby and up to 30 minutes after birth.

67. Assessment of the placenta should include (a) examination of membranes: a missing section may indicate retention of a piece of membrane in the uterus, and vessels traversing the membranes may indicate placenta succenturiate; (b) inspection of the umbilical cord for number of vessels, insertion site, and abnormalities, such as knots; and (c) inspection of the placenta for missing cotyledons, infarcts, and/or areas of calcification, and overall size and weight.

68. (a) Pitocin promotes rhythmic uterine contractions and assists in preventing uterine bleeding in the early postpartum time. (b) Assess maternal BP. See "Drug Guide: Oxytocin (Pitocin)." in Chapter 27.

69. (a) First stage: 8 hours. (b) Second stage: 1 hour 10 minutes. (c) Third stage: 15 minutes. (d) Fourth stage: began at 5:25 PM and lasted until 7:25 or 9:25 PM (2 to 4 hours)

70. See text, Table 24–7: Normal Progress, Psychologic characteristics, and Nursing Support During First and Second Stages of Labor, see Chapter 22.

71. c 72. c 73. a 74. a 75. b 76. b
77. c 78. a 79. b 80. b 81. b

82. When the uterus is not firmly contracting, the muscles become soft and blood collects in the uterus. A boggy uterus needs to be gently massaged until it is firm.

83. Comfort measures include cold pack to perineum, positioning, and pain medications if needed.

84. At the end of the recovery period the vital signs should be stable; the uterine fundus is in the midline, is firm, and is at the level of the umbilicus or 1 to 2 fingerbreadths below; the perineum is not excessively swollen or bruised; the episiotomy is not excessively swollen or bruised; and the skin edges are well approximated. If the woman has had regional anesthesia, she has usually regained sensation in the affected parts. In some hospitals, the recovery period does not end until the new mother has voided.

85. (a) First stage: Hypoxia of uterine muscle cells during contractions, stretching of the lower uterine segment and cervix, dilatation of the cervix, and pressure on adjacent structures.
(b) Second stage: Hypoxia of contracting uterine muscle cells, distention of the vagina and perineum, and pressure on adjacent structures.
(c) Third stage: Uterine contractions and cervical dilatation as the placenta is expelled.

86. See text, p. 686.

87. (a) The woman is willing to receive medication; vital signs are stable. (b) The FHR is between 110 and 160 beats per minute, and no decelerations are present; the fetus exhibits normal movement; the fetus is at term; meconium staining is not present. (c) Contraction pattern is well established; the fetal presenting part is engaged; there is progressive descent of the fetal presenting part. No complications are present.

88. (a) Active phase; 4 cm; Queen cries out and is restless, repeatedly changes positions, blood pressure and pulse increased, FHR 140. (b) It is difficult to identify the three top nursing considerations that all nurses would agree on. However, we suggest that the top three would be to (1) assess the woman's history and present status to identify contraindications for administering analgesics, (2) determine that the woman is not hypotensive and fetal status is normal (FHR is in normal range with average variability and no variable or late decelerations), and (3) ensure that the ordered medication is appropriate and the dosage is within the expected range. The next two nursing considerations would be to provide client safety after administration (e.g., ensure that side rails on bed are up, assist with all movement from bed, place call bell within reach) and reassess the woman and her fetus approximately 15 minutes after IM injection and 5 minutes after IV administration to ensure normal effects and to identify quickly untoward effects. Were your top three within the top five that we selected? (c) Formulas:

$$\frac{\text{Have mg}}{\text{Have mL}} : : \frac{\text{Desired mg}}{\text{Desired Ml}}$$

$$\frac{100\ \text{mg}}{1\ \text{mL}} : : \frac{75\ \text{mg}}{x\ \text{mL}}$$

$$100\ x = 75\ \text{mg}$$

$$x = 0.75\ \text{mL}$$

$$\frac{\text{Desired}}{\text{Have}} \times 1 =$$

$$\frac{75\ \text{mg}}{100\ \text{mg}} \times 1 = 0.75\ \text{mL}$$

(d) Dorsogluteal: see Fundamentals textbook. Ventrogluteal: see Fundamentals textbook.

89. (a) In active labor, the physician or CNM may administer an epidural block. (b) In the second stage, the physician may administer a pudendal or local anesthetic.

90. Kim is in early labor. Without an established contraction pattern, the epidural could decrease her current contractions. Encourage Kim to use relaxation and breathing techniques. Review them with her. If she insists on medication, advise her that an intravenous pain medication would have less effect on the labor progress and would provide her with some relief.

91. *Actions:* The immediate assessment should include looking at the perineum and performing a sterile vaginal examination if the head is not already visible.
Actions: While placing your gloved hand on the perineum just under the vagina to provide support to the perineal tissues, ask Carmen to push once more. As soon as the baby's head is born, ask Carolyn to pant. The panting will allow you a moment to suction the baby's mouth with a bulb syringe and to check quickly for a nuchal cord.
Actions: The newborn can be placed on the maternal chest with skin to skin contact to promote warmth and bonding.
Findings: You will slide your finger up along the side of the baby's head to feel for a loop of umbilical cord around the baby's neck. If you find a

loop, bend your finger at the first digit (making a "hook") and gently slip the cord over the baby's head.

92. (a) abortion, (b) estimated date of birth, (c) electronic fetal monitor, (d) deceleration, (e) episiotomy, (f) fetal heart rate, (g) head circumference, (h) last menstrual period, (i) rhesus factor, (j) rupture of membranes, (k) vaginal birth after cesarean

Chapter 13

1. Anxiety and fear are associated with fear of outcome, fear of performance or questions regarding ability to tolerate labor, fear of being hurt, anxiety regarding past experiences in the woman's life, inadequate knowledge, and lack of support. Anxiety may affect the labor by adding to the discomfort of uterine contractions and general body distress, making support and encouragement more difficult to accept, and slowing the labor and birth process.

2. Women with depression can present with a variety of symptoms including sad mood, physical slowing, agitation, energy loss, feelings of worthlessness, sleep disturbances, difficulty thinking or concentrating, fatigue, and irritability.

3. A variety of nursing diagnoses may be selected, such as **Anxiety related to stress of the labor process; Fear related to unknown outcome of labor;** or perhaps **Deficient Knowledge related to labor and birth process and associated comfort measures.**

4. Hypertonic labor usually occurs in the early latent phase. The contractions are more frequent than expected. Duration is short, but the discomfort experienced is far and above that of normal labor. The woman frequently becomes fearful regarding the rest of labor, disappointed due to the amount of discomfort and lack of progress, and exhausted. Hypotonic labor occurs during the late active or transitional phase. It is also associated with failure to progress as the contractions decrease in frequency, duration, and intensity, and the fetal descent slows or stops. The laboring woman experiences discomfort, disappointment, anxiety, and stress.

5. *Failure to progress* is a term used to describe very slow or lacking cervical dilatation and effacement, slow or lack of fetal descent (measured as "station" 0), and/or uterine contractions that do not increase in frequency, duration, and intensity. Or uterine contractions

may be deemed "adequate," however, cervical dilatation, effacement, and/or fetal descent is not occurring.

6. A physician may use active management to increase the chances that labor and birth will occur in a timely fashion. This begins with an amniotomy, followed by timed vaginal examinations to ensure that cervical dilatation is occurring at a rate of at least 1 cm/hr for a nullipara and 1.5 cm/hr for a multipara. If cervical dilatation is not occurring at this rate, augmentation of labor with IV oxytocin (Pitocin) is begun.

7. The most important aspect of treatment is to rule out cephalopelvic disproportion. Once ruled out, IV oxytocin augmentation is usually started.

8. Precipitous labor is labor that begins and ends within 3 hours.

9. Treatment of a woman who has experienced precipitous labor will be to induce any subsequent births.

10. June 15

11. June 29

12. Postterm pregnancy is frequently associated with decreased amounts of amniotic fluid, which sets the stage for compression of the umbilical cord. When compression of the cord is present, a variable deceleration of the FHR occurs. Other problems may include meconium aspiration and intrauterine growth restriction.

13. d, e   14. f, g   15. a   16. b, c

17. (a) Frank breech, (b) complete breech, (c) single footling breech

18. The drawing should show the umbilical cord prolapsing down below the cervix.

19. (a) A prolapsed cord is susceptible to compression, which slows the blood flow to the fetus and results in a slowing of the FHR and variable decelerations. The fetus is not being perfused in an adequate manner and is at risk. (b) You would feel a pulsating cord. You must keep your examining fingers against the fetal presenting part and exert slight pressure upward to relieve pressure on the cord. Have the woman put on her call light; once assistance arrives, they can apply the fetal monitor to assess the effectiveness of your intervention. Usually a cesarean birth must occur rapidly to maximize the outcome for the fetus. (c) See Figure 13–5 on p. 255 of answer key.

20. Abruptio placentae is separation of the placenta before birth of the fetus. The types are marginal, central, and complete.

21. Placenta previa is implantation of the placenta in the lower uterine segment or down over the internal cervical os. The placenta precedes the fetus. The types are low-lying, marginal, and complete.

22. b, d, f   23. c, e, f   24. a, d

25. See text, pp. 741–745.

26. No vaginal exam. In doing an exam, you may puncture one of the cotyledons and precipitate bleeding.

27. Risk factors include obesity, increased maternal glucose levels (gestational and pregestational diabetes), postterm pregnancy, multiparity, previous macrosomic infant, excessive weight gain, and maternal birth weight.

28. Shoulder dystocia

29. **Risk for Injury to Fetus related to trauma during the birth process; Risk for Infection related to traumatized tissue secondary to maternal tissue damage during birth; Deficient Knowledge related to lack of information about the implications and possible problems associated with a macrosomic baby.**

30. (a) The following criteria should be present before an external cephalic version is done: a single fetus (multiple gestation fetuses may become entangled); the fetal breech is not engaged (engagement increases the difficulty of the version); intact amniotic membranes and adequate amount of fluid (diminished amounts of fluid make the fetus hard to move and may cause cord compression); fetal well-being should be evident as demonstrated by a reassuring FHR pattern and reactive NST. (b) See text, pp. 759–762. (c) Some occult bleeding may occur during the version, and the woman could become sensitized at this time. (d) Pertinent areas to cover in discharge teaching include the following: being aware of uterine contractions and the possible beginning of labor, leakage of clear fluid from the vagina (amniotic fluid), increased or decreased fetal movement (may be associated with fetal stress), vaginal bleeding (may be associated with placental bleeding), the reason for administering Rh immune globulin (RhoGAM) if it was given, and the name and phone number of her physician in case there are further questions.

31. Indications for induction of labor include previous precipitous labor, postterm pregnancy, preexisting maternal disease (diabetes, preeclampsia), premature rupture of membranes (PROM), chorioamnionitis, fetal demise, IUGR, and mild abruptio placentae.

32. A positive CST means that late decelerations are present with uterine contractions. In this case, inducing labor would compromise the fetus.

33. Additional contraindications include client refusal, placenta previa, abnormal fetal presentation, prolapsed cord, prior classic uterine incision, active genital herpes, and CPD.

34. The Bishop score describes characteristics of the cervix and fetal position and assigns a score to different findings. The higher the score, the more likely that labor is ready to occur. A score of 3 would not be conducive to successful induction at this time. A score of 9 or more is compatible with successful induction.

35. The correct answer is 6 mL/hour. To compute this problem you need to start with the following facts:

$$1 \text{ mL Pitocin} = 10 \text{ units}$$
$$1 \text{ unit} = 1000 \text{ milliunits}$$
$$10 \text{ units} = 10{,}000 \text{ milliunits}$$
$$\frac{10{,}000 \text{ milliunits}}{1000 \text{ mL}} = \frac{x}{1 \text{ mL}}$$
$$x = 10 \text{ milliunits/mL of IV fluid}$$

There are 60 minutes in an hour, and you want 1 milliunit/min; 60 min × 1 milliunit/min = 60 milliunit/hr. To obtain milliliters per hour:

$$\frac{10 \text{ milliunits}}{1 \text{ mL}} = \frac{60 \text{ milliunits}}{x \text{ mL}}$$
$$10x = 60$$
$$x = 6 \text{ mL/hr}$$

   Did you arrive at the correct answer? This problem requires a lot of thought, but it is important to be able to calculate Pitocin infusion rates so that the client's safety can be maintained.

36. Signs of water intoxication include nausea, vomiting, hypotension, tachycardia, and cardiac arrhythmia.

37. Immediately before increasing the rate of intravenous Pitocin infusion, you must assess the following: maternal blood pressure and pulse, uterine contractions (frequency, duration, intensity), FHR (deviant patterns, variability), and fetal response (excessive activity).

38. The problems that might occur in response to a Pitocin induction include tetanic contractions, late or variable decelerations in FHR, a significant increase or decrease in maternal blood pressure or pulse, and signs of water intoxication if an electrolyte-free solution is used.

39. The sample fetal monitoring strip provides the following information: (a) The FHR baseline is 140 for the 8-minute segment. It is best to assess a 10-minute segment to accurately determine the baseline. (If you caught this point, congratulations. You had to know the definition of an FHR baseline and correctly count the spaces to realize that only 8 minutes are depicted.) (b) variability is present. (c) The variability is moderate. (d) Accelerations are not evident. (e) The contraction frequency is every 3 minutes. (f) The contraction duration is 60–75 seconds. (g) No. The infusion rate should not be advanced because "good" contractions have been achieved.

40. The strip indicates severe problems. (a) The immediate nursing actions would include discontinuing the Pitocin infusion and turning on the main IV line; turning the mother on her left side; starting oxygen administration at 6 to 10 L/min; notifying the physician; and anticipating preparations for effecting an immediate birth. (b) The strip showed severe late decelerations with minimal variability and tetanic contractions every $1^1/_2$ minutes lasting 80 to 90 seconds.

41. (a) Amniotomy is done to release amniotic fluid and allow the fetal presenting part (usually the occiput) to press more firmly on the cervix. This is thought to hasten labor. (b) First, the FHR should be assessed immediately after the membranes have been ruptured. The rationale for this action is that the umbilical cord may wash down through the cervix as the amniotic fluid escapes. As pressure is exerted on the cord, the fetal blood supply may be compromised. Second, you need to assess the amniotic fluid for amount, color, and odor.

42. (a) Greenish color is probably meconium staining, although presence of a foul odor could indicate infection. (b) Reddish color indicates that blood is present in the amniotic fluid. (c) Foul odor is associated with an infection in the amniotic fluid.

43. See answer at end of answer key on pp. 257–258.

44. The procedure is set up and administered in the same manner; however, response to the IV oxytocin is usually much quicker because uterine contractions are already occurring. The same assessments must be made.

45. Augmentation would be contraindicated in the following instances: in the presence of fetal distress, with strong suggestions of CPD, with hypertonic uterine contraction pattern, in the presence of placenta previa, and with multiple gestation. It is questionable with vaginal birth following cesarean birth.

46. You will need to call the obstetrician and inform her or him of the contraindications you have found. Perhaps the physician was unaware of the presence of the contraindications. If the physician persists in ordering the augmentation, ask what it is about the contraindications that you are not clear on and how it will still be safe for the client. Perhaps there is information that you do not have. If the contraindications persist, you will need to clearly explain that it is outside of your agency policy and you will not be able to do it as it violates your agency standards and your standard of nursing practice. You will need to chart your conversation clearly in the client record, and discuss this with your chain of command at this time.

47. (a) The Bishop score is 4; One point each for 1 to 2 cm dilatation, −2 station, moderate cervical consistency, and midposition of the cervix. Effacement of 30% equals 0 points. (b) Dinoprostone (Cervidil) is a prostaglandin gel that can be inserted into the vagina. Prostaglandin gel softens and effaces the cervix (see text for "Drug Guide: Dinoprostone Cervidil").

48. Signs and symptoms of twins include visualization of more than one gestational sac during ultrasound examination early in pregnancy, fundal height that exceeds the expected growth rate, and auscultation of two fetal heartbeats at least 10 beats per minute apart in rate.

49. Antepartal complications may include physical discomfort, dyspnea on exertion, preeclampsia, urinary tract infections, backaches, preterm labor, placenta previa, abruptio placentae, prolapsed cord, and hemorrhage during birth and postpartum.

50. Treatment plan will include areas such as increased nutritional intake, increased rest, and increased antepartal monitoring (visits, antepartal testing).

51. Implications for the fetuses may include inadequate nourishment of one fetus during gestation; premature labor, with associated problems of respiratory distress syndrome; difficulty in evaluating whether the second fetus can be born vaginally if the first fetus is born breech; interlocked fetuses; and slow or interrupted labor because of overstretching of the uterus.

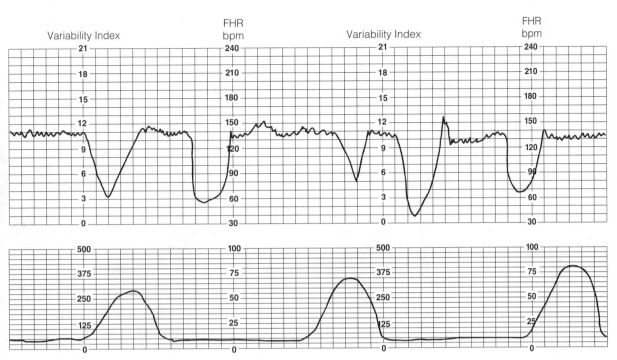

Figure 13–5

52. If one fetus exhibits problems, treatment must be initiated quickly in the same manner as it would if only one fetus were present.

53. Nonreassuring fetal status would be indicated by any of the following: loss of variability, severe late or variable decelerations, severe bradycardia, meconium staining in a vertex presentation, cessation of movement, or hyperactive fetal movement.

54. (a) postpartal bleeding and hemorrhage.
    (b) This occurs because of overstretching of the uterus and inadequate uterine contractions following birth.

55. 2000

56. Backache from increased weight in uterus and back strain, difficulty breathing from increased pressure upward on the diaphragm, and increased edema in feet, ankles, and legs due to increased pressure on vessels on lower extremities. See text for self-care measures.

57. Esophageal atresia that diminishes or prevents fetal swallowing may be identified by ultrasound. Kidney disorders that affect the fetal kidney output may be identified by ultrasound. Maternal diabetes, which affects the fetal urine output, is identified by maternal testing.

58. The uterus decompressed in size rapidly with the loss of a great amount of amniotic fluid. This may precipitate a change in the size of the uterus and the placenta may separate.

59. Oligohydramnios is defined as a severely decreased amount of concentrated amniotic fluid.

60. Variable decelerations, due to inadequate fluid that allows the umbilical cord to float without compression.

61. There is a decreased amount of fluid swallowed and urine produced and excreted by the fetus.

62. An amnioinfusion is a technique by which approximately 250 to 300 mL of warmed, sterile, saline or lactated Ringer's solution is introduced into the uterine cavity after membranes have ruptured (spontaneously or by amniotomy). The desired effect is to instill an adequate amount of fluid in order to relieve any pressure on the umbilical cord, which is indicated by the cessation of variable decelerations.

63. Another nursing intervention would be to change the woman's position.

64. During each variable deceleration, the fetus may be stressed and may release meconium into the amniotic fluid, which stains the fluid a light blackish green. With continued fetal stress, a larger amount of meconium may be released, making the amniotic fluid thicker and more discolored. Aspiration of the meconium-stained fluid can cause meconium aspiration pneumonitis after birth.

65. You should suspect a breech presentation.

66. When the fetus is in a breech presentation, there may be a release of meconium due to the

pressures occurring during contractions. In this instance, the release of meconium would most likely be viewed as physiologic. However, the possibility of fetal distress must be considered.

When there is evidence of meconium staining of the amniotic fluid during labor, the birth team needs to be prepared to remove secretions from the newborn's naso-oropharynx immediately after birth. Suction is frequently used to remove these secretions. In the case of a breech presentation, the newborn will be suctioned as soon as the head is born. In vertex presentation, the naso-oropharynx is suctioned as soon as the head appears, and before the first breath is taken, so that the secretions are not drawn into the lungs with the first breath. The vocal cords will be visualized with a laryngoscope. If meconium is seen, suctioning will be done. Aspiration of meconium can result in meconium aspiration pneumonia in the early neonatal period.

67. The maternal pelvis is greatly diminished in size. She will most likely need to have a cesarean birth.

68. Pelvic measurements would be obtained during antenatal care; while in labor, a clinical pelvimetry or x-ray pelvimetry may be done.

69. A TOL may be attempted in an effort to avoid an unnecessary cesarean birth. The woman would be induced or would come in when labor occurs and her progress would be closely watched in terms of uterine contractions, fetal status, and especially fetal descent.

70. Cervical dilatation in a primigravida is approximately 1.2 cm/hr; 1.5 cm/hr in a multigravida.

71. Fetal descent should be progressive from −3 to 0 and then +1 to +4 for vaginal birth.

72. Failure of cervix to dilate, failure of fetal descent, maternal pushing for greater than 2 hr (primigravida) or 3 hr (multigravida).

73. A gestation with a very large baby or a malposition (such as brow) that is larger than the maternal pelvis will accommodate. If the subsequent fetus is smaller, a vaginal birth may be possible.

74. Indications include maternal heart disease, maternal exhaustion, and fetal stress or distress.

75. Complete dilatation of the cervix, known fetal station and position, ruptured membranes.

76. See text, p. 777.

77. Maternal risks include lacerations of the birth canal and perineum and increased bleeding.

Fetal/neonatal risks include caput succedaneum or cephalhematoma, facial bruising, swelling or abrasions, and transient facial paralysis.

78. Nursing interventions that are necessary during a forceps-assisted birth include the following: Explain the procedure to the woman and her support person. Encourage the woman to maintain her breathing pattern during application of the forceps. (Panting may help to relieve the "need to push" sensation that she will feel as the forceps are applied.) Monitor the FHR continuously. Monitor contractions. Inform the physician when a contraction begins and ends, because he or she will exert downward pressure on the forceps during a contraction. Provide support to the woman throughout the process. Ensure that adequate resuscitation equipment is available and in working order before the birth. After birth, assess the newborn for Apgar score; facial bruising, swelling, abrasions, and/or paralysis; signs of cerebral trauma; and movement of arms (to detect paralysis).

79. The bruising and swelling will slowly go away, and there will not be any lasting effects for their baby.

80. (a) The vacuum extractor is devised to apply negative pressure on the fetal occiput so that traction may be applied to the extractor and the fetus is assisted in the birth. (b) The negative pressure that builds up in the cup draws the fetal scalp up and edema forms in the tissues. The "chignon" is an area of swelling (caput) that is the size and shape of the extractor cup. (c) The parents need to know the reason the extractor is needed, and the expected effects, benefits, and risks for both the mother and fetus/newborn. The mother's permission needs to be verbally obtained.

81. (a) Cleanse the maternal abdomen from the umbilicus downward to just over the symphysis. (b) The indwelling bladder catheter is inserted in the same manner as for other adults, with the exception that identification of the urethral meatus may be more difficult because of swelling of the vulvar tissues and that actual insertion of the catheter may take more pressure because the fetal head is down against the vulvar tissues. (c) See text, pp. 784–785.

82. 37.5

83. See text, pp. 783–784.

84. See text, pp. 783–784.

85. If your teaching has been effective, Kirsten will understand the need to move her legs frequently

during the recovery phase, she will take deep breaths and cough while splinting her abdomen with a pillow; she will ask for pain medication when she feels she needs it; she will cooperate with the turning and changing of position every 2 hours; and she will cooperate with ambulation to facilitate return of bowel motility.

86. The father's comfort can be enhanced by answering any questions that he has, providing information regarding the cesarean birth, and describing ways in which he may want to be involved. See further discussion in text, p. 786.

87. Vaginal birth after cesarean (VBAC) can be attempted after one previous cesarean if there are no contraindications. Once a woman has more than one cesarean birth, VBAC is contraindicated and a repeat cesarean is indicated. More than one cesarean increases the risk of a uterine rupture.

88. (a) Contraindications would include a previous classic uterine incision, inability to perform a cesarean within 30 minutes, and client refusal. (b) Becky needs to present with a history of not more than two previous cesareans. The previous uterine incisions should not be classic incisions. During labor, the maternal assessment would include vital signs for early detection of hemorrhage, uterine contraction pattern for normal contraction characteristics, and fetus for reassuring FHR pattern.

89. Of the three choices, "insufficient data" was the correct choice. The abdominal incision and the uterine incision do not necessarily match. The only way to validate the type of uterine incision is to review the surgical record of the first cesarean birth. If the uterine incision is a "classic" incision, a VBAC is usually contraindicated. If the type of uterine incision cannot be determined, many obstetricians would recommend a cesarean for any succeeding pregnancies.

90. (a) This is a very difficult situation. Anna deserves straight, honest information. You might say something like, "I'm very sorry, Anna. I did not hear your baby's heartbeat. Your doctor is on the way. May I sit with you while we wait?"

As a student, you may have fears that you will not hear the FHR and mistakenly think the baby is dead. In reality, you will be assessing FHR with your instructor or with birthing room staff. When you are just learning to listen to FHR and you either are not able to hear the FHR at all or are not sure what you are hearing, you might say

to the nurse, "I'm not as experienced as you in listening to the FHR, and I'm not sure what I'm hearing. Would you listen to it now, please?" (b) Ultrasound

91. See text, Chapter 37.

92. Comments such as a and b that devalue the baby's worth or minimize the loss are insensitive. Even if Nadine conceives again, that baby will not replace the one she lost. Even though the baby had a birth defect, the comment suggests she is better off losing the baby than having a baby with Down Syndrome. Answer c conveys empathy and compassion. Many need support after a fetal loss. Because each woman grieves differently, some women may not want visitors while in the hospital, but others may desire support from family and friends. Answer d should not be assumed. Instead, the nurse should ask the mother about her personal preferences.

93. The responses she is experiencing are normal aspects of the grieving process. Everyone experiences grief differently and their own pace. You should assure Nadine and offer support. You should make sure Nadine has adequate support services in place. Although these reactions are a normal grief response, you need to make sure she is not experiencing any suicidal thoughts or feelings. You should provide referrals for counseling and support groups.

94. (a) Artificial rupture of membranes; (b) biparietal diameter; (c) cephalopelvic disproportion; (d) cesarean section; (e) disseminated intravascular coagulation; (f) hemolysis, elevated liver enzymes, low platelets; (g) intrauterine fetal death; (h) meconium staining of amniotic fluid; (i) Pitocin; (j) sterile vaginal examination; (k) trial of labor; (l) vaginal birth after cesarean

43. Based on the case scenario, the most pertinent responses could include:

Collaborative problems: 1. Potential complications of magnesium sulfate therapy
2. Magnesium toxicity

Nursing diagnosis: Breathing Pattern, ineffective

Defining characteristics:
Decreasing respiratory rate, resp. rate less than 12 breaths/min

Altered chest excursion

Goal/Evaluation Criteria	Nursing Activities	Evaluation of Goal
NOC language: demonstrates uncompromised Respiratory Status: Ventilation as evidenced by depth of respirations, symmetric chest expansion, adventitious breath sounds.	**Assessments:** • Monitor resp. rate, chest excursion • Monitor for pallor and cyanosis **Interventions:**	• Respiratory rate 14 breaths min, equal chest excursion • No adventitious sounds • Chest expansion symmetric
OR **Client/husband will:**	**NIC Priority Intervention** Airway management	
demonstrate respiratory rate greater than 11	• Facilitating patency of airway passages	
have absence of adventitious breath sounds	• Positioning • TCDB every hour Respiratory monitoring • Monitor rate, rhythm, depth & effect of respirations **Other Nursing Activities**	

Chapter 14

1. (a) Mechanical: The baby's passage through the birth canal fosters removal of fluid from the lungs and throat. The chest recoil results in the taking in of air. When air is expelled against a partially closed glottis, it fosters an increase in pressure within the chest and opens alveoli.
(b) Chemical stimuli: Increase in P_{CO_2} and decrease in oxygen triggers respiratory center. Prolonged asphyxia acts as a depressant.
(c) Thermal stimuli: Decrease in environment temperature stimulates skin nerve endings and rhythmic breathing. (d) Sensory stimuli: Tactile (thorough drying), auditory, and visual.

2. The newborn's cardiovascular system accomplishes the following anatomic and physiologic alterations during the transition from fetal to neonatal circulation: increase in aortic pressure and decrease in venous pressure as a result of loss of the placenta; increased systemic pressure and decreased pulmonary artery pressure due to decreased pulmonary circulatory resistance and vasodilation; closure of the ductus venosus and foramen ovale; and closure of the ductus arteriosus, which increases blood flow in the pulmonary vascular system.

3. a

4. Physiologic jaundice usually appears about the second or third day of life. Jaundice is the yellow color that can be seen in the newborn's eyes and skin. It comes from normal breakdown of RBCs and the liver's decreased ability to process and excrete bilirubin, which results in a temporary buildup of bilirubin in the blood and fatty tissue under the skin. Usually gone by 10th to 14th day of life. The time of onset is important to note because it will help you differentiate jaundice that is considered pathologic when it occurs at birth or within the first 24 hours after birth.

5. See text, p. 814–815.

6. a   7. a

8. To anticipate possible physiologic problems and establish an individualized plan of newborns and their families.

9. (a) 38, (b) 39

10. AGA, see text, pp. 819–820.

11. (a) 97.5F to 99F (36.4C to 37.3C) axillary; (b) 120 to 160 beats per minute (100 asleep, 180 crying); (c) 30 to 60 breaths per minute; (d) 80 to 60/45 to 40 mmHg

12. (a) 3405 g (7 lb, 8 oz caucasian, varies with ethnicity); (b) 5 to 10.

13. Small fluid intake, increased volume of meconium stooling, fluid shifts, and increased urination.

14. a

15. See text, p. 830, Figure 29–15.

16. Place infant flat on the back with legs extended as much as possible; if breech birth, remeasure when legs are no longer in the in utero breech position.

17. 50 cm (20 in.), range 45 to 55 cm (18 to 22 in.)

18. a   19. b

20. See text, pp. 838–840.

21. See text, pp. 848–858.

22. c   23. c

24. Answers may include the following: yawn, blink, cough/sneeze, gag, withdrawal from painful stimuli.

25. See text, pp. 833, 835, 837, 840–843.

26. Decreased peripheral circulation, which results in vasomotor instability and capillary stasis, can often be seen as acrocyanosis.

Chapter 15

1. As the newborn nurse, you should ascertain the following essential areas of information from the birthing room nurse: previously identified perinatal risk factors; problems occurring during labor and birth, such as signs of fetal distress or maternal problems (abruptio placentae, preeclampsia, and prolapse of the cord, all of which compromise the fetus in utero); medications given to the mother during labor or given to the newborn in the immediate postbirth period; the baby's Apgar scores; airway clearance; resuscitative measures administered to the newborn; elimination during the postbirth period (did the newborn void or pass meconium in the birthing room?); vital signs, general condition, activity level, and neurologic status; ability to feed; and evidence of complications. If you identified these areas, you have a basis for identifying significant potential problems for the newborn. These areas of information provide a database from which to make continued careful and significant observations and nursing diagnoses during the transitional period.

2. Nursing actions that you would perform during the admission process and continue for the first 4 hours after birth would be assessing for any signs of neonatal distress: noting vital signs (including blood pressure in some agencies); measuring weight; measuring length; taking head and chest circumference measurements; administering prophylactic medications; scoring for gestational age; and doing blood work (hematocrit and heel-stick glucose) at 4 hours of age. In addition, many institutions do a general head-to-toe admission physical. Other institutions may also do stomach aspirations; however, this procedure is controversial and should not be done until the newborn is stable, because it can cause bradycardia and apnea.

3. Absence of normal intestinal bacterial flora needed to synthesize vitamin K results in low levels of vitamin K. This creates a transient blood coagulation deficiency between the second and fifth day of life. 1 mg IM.

4. *Actions:* Immediately after Prakash's birth, you would dry him off, assess the heart and respiratory rates, determine the 1- and 5-minute Apgar scores, and then do a quick physical assessment for congenital anomalies.

   Actions: Place Prakash skin to skin with his mother. Cover them both with a warm blanket to assist in maintaining his temperature. Assist Prakash to suckle at the breast, and provide any support Prakash and his mom may need to facilitate the bonding process.

5. c

6. (a) Ophthalmic neonatorum, (b) *Neisseria gonorrhoeae*

7. Answers may include 0.5% erythromycin or 1% tetracycline.

8. Polycythemia, increase fluid intake; anemia, observe for any respiratory distress; jaundice, assess need for phototherapy; hypoglycemia, observe for signs of jitteriness and temperature instability and initiate early feedings (breast milk or glucose water).

9. A possible nursing diagnosis would be **Ineffective Airway Clearance.** You would immediately aspirate the mouth and nasal pharynx with a bulb syringe, holding the newborn with his head down and neck extended to facilitate drainage as you aspirate the mucus. If you also recognize an increase in mucus production during the second period of reactivity, you are becoming alert and prepared to intervene in this very real problem.

10. Neonatal assessments following transition should include (a) vital signs, (b) weight, (c) stool pattern, (d) voiding pattern, (e) caloric and fluid intake, and (f) status of umbilical cord.

11. Urine is straw-colored and odorless; may be cloudy with mucus strands; will have increased specific gravity and decreased output until oral intake increases.

12. Check chart and see whether Ryan voided at birth. Assess for adequacy of fluid intake, bladder distention, restlessness, and signs of discomfort. Notify appropriate clinical personnel.

13. Within 12 to 24 hours or at least by 48 hours of life. First stools are meconium, which are thick, tarry, and dark green-black.

14. The nursing diagnosis: **Health-Related Behaviors related to lack of information about breastfeeding correctly** might apply. Ms. Montoya is obviously eager to be successful but has many unanswered questions. Her statement, even though not phrased as a request, was her way of reaching out and asking for assistance.

15. See text, pp. 906–908.

16. b   17. d

18. See text pp. 910–913.

19. Because women are often discharged within 24 hours of birth, it is difficult to effectively complete infant care teaching. You can help reinforce Ms. Montoya's learning by presenting material in different ways (verbal instruction followed by practice, for example, or by showing a videotape followed by discussion). You can then reinforce positive behaviors. For example, if you observe Ms. Montoya using the football hold, you might say, "I think it's really wise of you to try using the different feeding positions. Can you feel the difference in the suction when your baby is in this position?" When she is ready to leave, it is always helpful to provide handouts with specific information so the new mother will have a practical reference at home. By the same token, Ms. Montoya may find it helpful to have the phone number of the mother-baby unit so she can call someone if questions arise.

20. Your teaching plan will have been effective if Helena is able to successfully breastfeed her infant and demonstrate the techniques you have covered. For the cognitive content covered, you can ask Helena to describe to you the information you have shared. You can then discuss it briefly to learn whether she understands it fully.

21. d

22. It is not uncommon for newborns to have decreased intake and weight loss in the first week of life. By the end of the first week, the newborn should regain weight and start gaining weight at about 1 oz/day for the first 6 months. Intake should not exceed 32 oz/day. Ascertain how much Christy is eating and encourage her mother to offer the bottle at least every 3 to 4 hours.

23. b   24. a, c

25. Based on information in Chapters 29 and 30, formulate an informative and supportive response to these mothers' questions and concerns during parenting classes.

26. Ascertain whether the parents have any questions and whether they have signed the permit based on information; gather equipment and prepare Ryan by removing diaper; provide for topical anesthetic before procedure and pain medication before and after as needed; provide comfort measures during and after procedure; assess for adequacy of voiding; and assess for bleeding.

27. d

28. Cleanse the penis daily, but do not attempt to retract the foreskin.

29. c   30. a   31. d

32. Essential components of a newborn discharge teaching program would include bathing (skin, scalp, and nail care), eye and ear care, nasal suctioning (use of a bulb syringe), cord care, circumcision care or care of the uncircumcised male infant, care of female genitalia, diapering, positioning and handling, establishing a feeding schedule versus feeding on demand, burping, pumping the breasts and supplemental feeding for breastfed infants, formula preparation, introduction to solids (what, when, why), providing vitamin supplements, stooling and voiding patterns, sleep patterns, self-soothing methods, clothing, neonatal behavioral changes that may occur after discharge, observation for signs of illness, use of the thermometer, testing for phenylketonuria, administration of hepatitis B and pediatric follow-up.

33. a

34. See text, pp. 883, 885.

35. a

36. See "Developing Cultural Competence" on text p. 880.

37. (a) abdominal circumference, (b) brown adipose tissue, (c) chest circumference, (d) head circumference, (e) phenylketonuria

Chapter 16

1. Answers may include exposure to environmental hazards; low socioeconomic level; preexisting maternal condition such as diabetes, age, or

parity; gestational diseases; and pregnancy complications.

2. Baby Joey's gestational age is 36 to 37 weeks, which places him as being preterm, and his weight of 1500 g places him below the 10th percentile for weight. His GA and weight classify him as a preterm SGA newborn. Based on this classification, you would want to watch Joey for the potential problems of hypothermia, respiratory distress, hypoglycemia, hypocalcemia, and polycythemia.

3. postterm

4. preterm

5. large for gestational age

6. small for gestational age

7. c

8. Answers may include primiparity or grandmultiparity, small stature, preeclampsia, substance abuse, lack of prenatal care, smoking, and age less than 16 or greater than 40 years.

9. a

10. b, c, d

11. IDM babies are LGA and macrosomic and may be plethoric: they have large placentas and umbilical cords.

12. See text, p. 939.

13. Serum glucose levels on cord blood, hourly for first 4 hours, then every 4 hours until stable.

14. 40

15. b

16. Early detection and ongoing monitoring of signs of hypoglycemia and polycythemia; provision of adequate caloric intake with breast milk or formula and infusion of glucose as ordered.

17. d   18. d   19. F   20. T

21. F   22. T

23. b

24. Answers may include the following: maternal disease such as cardiac or renal disease, diabetes, preeclampsia, cervical incompetence, infections; substance abuse, multiple fetuses, fetal infections, hydramnios; low socioeconomic level, poor prenatal care; history of preterm births.

25. b

26. The three initial assessments you should make on the arrival of a preterm newborn in the nursery area are observation of signs of respiratory distress, core temperature determination to assess whether hypothermia or cold stress will complicate this infant's course, and gestational

age determination to identify other potential problems. You may have identified other areas, but these are the essential ones. Refer to your textbook if you had any difficulty identifying the initial needs of the preterm newborn.

27. b   28. a   29. d

30. See text, pp. 945–948.

31. b

32. See text, pp. 948–950 and Procedure 32–1.

33. Nursing assessments of Mary's tolerance of gavage feedings would include observing for any degree of abdominal distention during or after the feeding; a formula residual of less than 1 mL before the next feeding; lack of regurgitation; and no apnea, bradycardia, cyanosis, or color changes. A program of alternate gavage and nipple feeding is recommended to decrease the possibility of fatigue during feeding.

34. d

35. See text, pp. 957–959.

36. Some complications associated with cocaine-exposed infants include poor state organization and decreased interactive behaviors, congenital malformations, withdrawal, and motor development problems.

37. See text, p. 966, Table 32–4.

38. b   39. c   40. b

41. Needs may include comfort measures such as swaddling and small frequent feedings.

42. c

43. See text, pp. 972–974.

44. d

45. (a) acquired immunodeficiency syndrome, (b) alcohol-related birth defects, (c) fetal alcohol syndrome, (d) infant of diabetic mother, (e) infant of substance-abusing mother, (f) intrauterine growth restriction, (g) large for gestational age, (h) small for gestational age

Chapter 17

1. d

2. (a) Meconium aspiration syndrome (MAS); (b) oropharynx, then nasopharynx are suctioned via low-pressure wall suction; (c) if thick meconium is present, clinician may visualize glottis and suction meconium from trachea.

3. If you answered "no," you were correct. Celeste is not a candidate for further resuscitation because of her vigorous crying after birth, no signs of respiratory distress, and the thin nature of the meconium-stained amniotic fluid.

Vigorous resuscitation with intubation is avoided in this situation as it may do more harm to the baby.

Your most pressing nursing goal is to dry off the baby and continue assessment of respiratory function.

4. Vigorous suctioning can stimulate the vagus nerve and cause bradycardia.

5. (a) 15 to 25, (b) 40 to 60

6. Brian probably has narcotic depression; you would give Narcan and continue ventilatory support.

7. c 8. d 9. c, d.

10. Congratulations if you scored Tricia's respiratory distress as 6. This is based on nasal flaring = 1, lower chest retractions = 1, xiphoid retractions = 1, chest lag on inspiration = 1, and expiratory grunting = 2. Tricia is having significant respiratory distress. Based on her small size and early gestational age, she is using large amounts of energy in her work of breathing and will exhaust her supply of surfactant.

11. Tricia's history of preterm birth, a low Apgar score (hypoxic insult), and a low core temperature (cold stress) are all contributing factors to her development of respiratory distress syndrome.

12. See Nursing Care Plan. The Newborn with Respiratory Distress Syndrome in Chapter 33.

13. See text, p. 996, Table 33–2.

14. c

15. The metabolic effects of cold stress include competition for albumin binding sites by increased nonesterified fatty acids, causing increased free circulating bilirubin; increased incidence of hypoglycemia resulting from glucose being used for thermogenesis; pulmonary vasoconstriction in response to the release of norepinephrine; and increase in oxygen consumption and metabolic acidosis as the body burns brown fat deposits. If you were successful in identifying these changes, you will also be aware that these changes may create serious life-threatening problems for an at-risk infant.

16. c 17. a

18. Some of the causes are fetal-neonatal asphyxia, hypothermia, hypoglycemia, maternal use of sulfa, aspirin, intracranial hemorrhage, and Rh-negative hemolytic disease; total bilirubin greater than 15 mg/dL for term newborns; occurs within the first 24 hours.

19. d

20. Your assessment of developing jaundice may be affected by fluorescent nursery lights with pink tints, which mask jaundice; by blue walls and blue blankets; and by the basic pigmentation of the gumline in ethnic people of color.

21. a

22. *Analysis:* You remember that one of the criteria for differentiating physiologic jaundice from pathologic jaundice is the time of onset. Because Alice is less than 24 hours old, it leads you to think the jaundice is pathologic in nature. Breastfeeding jaundice usually does not start until after 3 days. Sepsis is a possibility and requires further investigation.

Actions: Your nursing actions would include checking Alice's chart and her mother's chart for risk factors. As you check these charts, you find that her mother received no prenatal care, and the blood typing was done on admission. Alice's perinatal history reveals that the birth was normal without trauma, asphyxiation, or delay of the cord clamping. Alice was scored as a term AGA newborn. You complete your physical assessment to determine the extent of the jaundice and any other significant clinical findings such as activity state and bruising.

Actions: Laboratory data that you would expect to be evaluated include indirect and direct bilirubin, blood typing, Coombs' test on Alice's blood, complete white count, and RBC smear.

23. c 24. b 25. a 26. b 27. d

28. Some causes are prematurity, passage through the birth canal, premature rupture of maternal membranes, immature immune system of newborn, and invasive procedures.

29. Answers may include gram-negative organisms (*E. coli, Enterobacter, Proteus, Klebsiella*) and gram-positive β-hemolytic streptococcus.

30. a

31. See text, pp. 1024–1027.

32. a

33. See text, pp. 1029–1032.

34. See text, pp. 1033–1034.

35. (a) Bronchopulmonary dysplasia, (b) meconium aspiration syndrome, (c) neutral thermal environment, (d) respiratory distress syndrome, (e) umbilical arterial catheterization

Chapter 18

1. See text, Chapter 34.

2. Stage 4 (after the birth of the placenta to 1 to 4 hours past birth).

3. Cuddling and holding the baby, talking to the baby, stroking movements, smiling, *en face* position, seeking out eye contact, making soothing noises, and asking questions about the baby are some examples.

4. Continue to provide opportunities for the parents to hold and interact with the baby. Complete any nursing activities while the baby is being held if at all possible, turn off the overhead lights to allow the baby to open its eyes, and encourage the parents in their activities.

5. b   6. d   7. b   8. c   9. b

10. (a) Postpartal chill is usually experienced immediately after birth. It is thought to be related to the emptying of the uterus, the rapid cardiovascular changes that are occurring, and emotional responses to birth. (b) Postpartal diaphoresis occurs on the day of birth or the first postpartum day. The body needs to shed extra fluid that has been retained during the pregnancy. The new mother may wake up in the night drenched with perspiration. (c) *Afterpains* is a term used to refer to the rhythmic uterine contractions that continue to occur after birth. The contractions are essential for involution to occur.

11. It is a time of enormous readjustment and readaptation to role, family, and self-image.

12. The term *postpartum blues* refers to a feeling of depression and weepiness that many mothers experience in the first few days after birth.

13. See text, pp. 1047–1048.

14. The following essential areas need to be included in your daily physical assessment of the postpartal client: vital signs; breasts, including nipples; fundus and abdomen; lochia; perineum (including the anus); elimination; lower extremities; nutritional status; activity level.

    If you listed most of these, you are well on your way to providing good nursing care for your clients. If you missed three or more, you need to refer back to the postpartum section in your textbook. Other areas that may be considered are discomfort level and sleep patterns.

15. Note softness or firmness, filling, and engorgement. If the woman is breastfeeding, note nipple soreness, cracking of nipples, and areas of firmness. This is also a good time to determine whether the mother does breast self-examinations and to provide teaching if she does not know how and desires to.

16. (a) To evaluate involution. (b) A full bladder may push the uterine fundus upward and to the maternal right side. The assessment will be inaccurate and palpating a full bladder will add to the mother's discomfort. Also, a woman with a full bladder is more likely to have heavier lochia. (c) Place the palm of your hand at the level of the umbilicus and cup it back toward the maternal spine. Feel for a rounded, firm object. (d) Usually recorded as the number of fingerbreadths above or below the umbilicus.

17. Up toward the umbilicus and in the midline.

18. Lochia rubra, moderate amount, without clots.

19. Per agency policy

20. As she lies on her back, lochia collects in the vagina. When she stands, the collected lochia is discharged. As long as the uterus is firm and in the midline and the flow is not more than moderate, she is fine.

21. lateral Sims'

22. Such as observe for hemorrhoids.

23. Bladder distention, amount of urine being voided, any difficulty or pain with voiding.

24. Whether she has had a bowel movement or not. What her normal bowel pattern is.

25. Teaching could include the following: dietary needs for maintaining stool patterns; need for rest, exercise, and adequate fluids. You can assess what the mother finds helpful to stimulate bowel movements.

26. To assess for bruising, edema, tenderness, redness, muscle strain, and thrombophlebitis.

27. By dorsiflexing the foot.

28. *Analysis:* You suspect that Ms. Sams's bladder is distended. You know that because the uterine ligaments are still stretched, a distended bladder can easily displace the uterus and cause it to appear higher in the abdomen. It may also keep the uterus from remaining firmly contracted.

    Analysis: You assist Ms. Sams to the bathroom so she can attempt to void. You place a "Johnny cap" under the seat of the commode so you can measure her output. You show her where the call light is, and you leave her in privacy to attempt to void.

    Analysis: You know that a distended bladder is common postpartally. You also know that pressure and trauma can reduce bladder sensitivity and tone. However, if Ms. Sams is not able to void, it may be necessary to catheterize her. You hope to avoid catheterization because of the associated risk of infection.

    Analysis: You employ nursing measures to assist Ms. Sams. You pour a measured amount of warm water slowly over her perineum while her wrist is resting in warm water. You also create a verbal picture of flowing water for her. You encourage her to use her other hand to massage her bladder.

Analysis: You are pleased that Ms. Sams has been able to void successfully. You decide to reassess her uterus to be certain it is now firm.

Analysis: The fact that Ms. Sams has been able to void two large amounts suggests that her bladder tone is adequate.

Analysis: You tell Ms. Sams that you think she is doing well. You point out that incomplete emptying of the bladder can lead to a boggy uterus and may also contribute to the development of a bladder infection. You ask her to monitor her next two or three voidings and report to the nurse if she feels that she is not emptying her bladder fully or if she begins voiding in small amounts.

Nice job! You made accurate assessments and employed nursing actions effectively. You also treated Ms. Sams like a responsible adult by explaining the situation and involving her in assuming responsibility for her own care.

29. Inquire about her usual eating habits and provide information regarding RDA if she desires.

30. Observe how the mother interacts with others: is she animated, does she smile, does she keep eye contact, is she able to ask for what she needs, is she hesitant or reticent with you or with specific family members? Remember that many of the characteristics just listed are culturally conditioned and therefore subjective, and careful follow-up is needed.

31. (a) Episiotomy Laceration: cold packs, sitz bath, sitting on a firm surface, spraying the area with warm water after urinating. (b) Hemorrhoids: witch hazel packs, Tucks, patting when drying after urinating. (c) Afterpains: warm packs, holding pillow against abdomen, lying on her stomach, analgesics.

32. The mother wears a firm bra and avoids any stimulation to the breasts. Engorgement occurs and then will slowly dissipate. It is uncomfortable for the mother.

33. (a) Assess her steadiness, dizziness, skin temperature and characteristics, skin color, BP, and pulse. (b) Need for cleansing the vulva and perineum after voiding with a spray bottle of warm water or something similar, patting with toilet paper instead of wiping, patting from front to back to decrease incidence of UTI, any measures to increase her comfort. (c) Make sure

she knows how to operate the emergency call button in the shower and stay in the room while she is in the shower. She is at the most risk of fainting at this time.

34. Answers may include the desire for this child, her support system, methods of coping, resources, life desire, and knowledge base.

35. By providing support, encouragement, and information as desired by the mother. Role modeling also is very helpful.

36. Sit down and listen to her. She is expressing feelings of sadness, frustration, and fear. Use reflective communication techniques and stay with her words. Avoid false reassurance and belittling comments. She needs to know she is being heard and understood and that these feelings are shared by many mothers.

37. The following are some suggestions for the Clarks: Enroll Tanner in a sibling class before the birth. Have Tanner come in for visits while in the birthing facility. Provide many opportunities for him to have special attention or activities, cuddle him, and introduce him to the new baby. Bring Tanner a gift or special treat from his new sister. Provide opportunities for caretaking and holding and introduction to the new role of big brother. Encourage role-playing with baby dolls.

38. The father or support person can be included more readily by encouraging him or her to visit whenever possible during the day or evening and to participate in infant care, encouraging him or her to come in for infant feeding, including him or her in parenting classes in the postpartal unit, being supportive of his or her efforts, providing time for any questions, and including him or her in all teaching.

These are just a few possibilities. You may have thought of others.

39. You should include information about her obstetric history, including the following: number of pregnancies, births, and abortions; significant prenatal problems and conditions; date and time of birth; medications given (anesthesia and analgesics); course of labor and birth (e.g., time of rupture of membranes, use of forceps, episiotomy, prolonged second stage); sex, Apgar score, and present condition of the infant, along with pertinent recovery room data; available support systems (in many agencies the mother's marital status has little relevance; the focus is on the support she has available to her); any existing problems or complaints (including

allergies to food or drugs); method of feeding the infant; teaching needs.

If you included most of this information, you are on the right track. If you included the physical aspects but neglected the support and teaching areas, you may find it helpful to review material related to psychologic adjustments and teaching needs during the early postpartal period.

40. (a) High on your list of priorities in planning Carla's physical care should be rest and comfort. With an 18-hour labor, you know she has been up all night and most of the preceding day. Her third-degree extension and hemorrhoids make comfort important, and meeting this need will enable her to rest more easily.

Because this is probably her first shower, safety is a fairly high priority, as it is with most women following birth. You should also use this time for postpartal teaching before she is discharged.

If you listed bladder or intestinal elimination as a high priority, you may wish to review your textbook.

It is always pertinent to assess a postpartal woman for hemorrhage, but because her fundus has remained firm, it would not be your highest priority. (b) You can assess Carla's attitude toward her child by unobtrusively observing her with her infant and by discussing the subject with her in an open, nonjudgmental way. Although her history suggests a possible bonding problem, it is not appropriate to jump to conclusions without further data. Frequently parents will express initial disappointment about a child's sex or behavior and then bond beautifully later.

41. Because of the incision, the mother needs careful, gentle assessment of her uterine fundus and a full surgical assessment.

42. (a) Patient-controlled analgesia is helpful for clients in that they can press the button for release of an analgesic agent as they need for comfort. (b) The PCA pump is set to deliver a specified amount of analgesic with each push of the button.

43. See text, p. 1095.

44. See text, p. 1095.

45. See Chapter 35, text, p. 1095.

46. It is important for LaTisha to know that the test is less accurate until there is an adequate intake of breast milk or formula. Although a test will be taken before discharge, the follow-up second test is essential.

Chapter 19

1. Answers include assessment, teaching, and counseling.

2. Typically only one or two postpartal visits are planned, long-term follow-up is not anticipated, and the scope of the visit is focused (on postpartal needs) rather than comprehensive.

3. See text, pp. 1104–1105.

4. Terminate the visit.

5. b

6. The newborn's skull bones are soft, and permanently flattened areas may develop if the infant lies consistently in one position.

7. Back position is recommended by American Academy of Pediatrics to reduce risk of sudden infant death syndrome (SIDS).

8. Sponge baths are recommended until the umbilical cord has fallen off and the site has healed (up to about 2 weeks).

9. See text, p. 1110.

10. axillary

11. F   12. T   13. F   14. F

15. T   16. F   17. T

18. See text, p. 111.

19. Answers may include restoring her physical condition, developing competence in caring for and meeting the needs of her newborn, establishing a relationship with her new child, and adapting to an altered lifestyle and family structure.

20. See text, pp. 1113–1115.

21. 6   22. 1   23. 1   24. 1

25. 6   26. 1   27. 6

28. Answers may include failure to cuddle or soothe the infant, failure to seek eye-to-eye contact, failure to call infant by name, failure to attain adequate supplies to care for the infant, calling infant by a nickname that promotes ridicule, inadequate infant weight gain, infant dirty and poorly kept, and severe diaper rash.

29. Based on the case scenario, the most pertinent responses could include:

Collaborative problems: 1. Development of cracked nipples

2. Signs and symptoms of mastitis

Nursing diagnosis: Pain

Defining characteristics:

Facial mask of pain, guarding or protective behaviors, grimacing

(Continued on page 266)

30. b   31. d   32. e   33. c   34. a

Goal/Evaluation Criteria	Nursing Activities	Evaluation of Goal
Client will: report decrease in nipple pain. have no nipple cracking present.	**Assessments:** • Inspect nipples for redness, cracking. **Interventions:** • Instruct in use of OTC analgesics. • Instruct mother in self-care measures. **Other Nursing Activities**	• Mother vocalized decreased pain and discomfort with breastfeeding. • No grimacing noted.

Chapter 20

1. (a) Greater than 500 mL in first 24 hours after birth; uterine atony, lacerations of genital tract, retained placental fragments. (b) After first 24 hours postbirth, retained placental fragments or membranes.

2. Joan is predisposed to early postpartal hemorrhage because of overdistention of the uterus, which is present with a full-term multiple pregnancy, and because of her precipitous labor.

3. See text, p. 1165, Table 38–2. Answers include the following: slow, steady, free flow of bleeding as assessed by pad counts or weighing peri-pads; boggy, soft fundus that does not stay contracted with massage and that expresses large clots; and changes in vital signs that reflect possible hypovolemia.

4. a

5. Early identification and management of uterine relaxation/atony and blood loss are high priorities. Another high priority is assisting Joan and her husband to deal with the anxiety over her bleeding.

6. Assess fundal height and firmness; administer methylergonovine maleate as ordered; have Joan empty her bladder frequently. If bleeding is profuse, give oxygen by mask, give medications, and assess effectiveness. Blood loss may cause anemia, so assess for pallor and fatigue, and check hematocrit. Encourage rest while facilitating maternal-infant attachment.

7. *Actions:* As you assess Carrie's episiotomy for redness, swelling, warmth, and intactness, you would also visualize and palpate her total perineal area to assess for hematoma development.

   Actions: Your nursing actions to improve comfort would include application of covered ice packs to decrease the swelling and discomfort. You may also use sitz baths to aid in fluid absorption and give analgesics as ordered and needed. You may also encourage her to void to avoid the need for catheterization. Careful observation and palpation of this site are essential so that you can assess any extension or enlargement of the hematoma. Frequent monitoring of vital signs every 15 min will enable you to assess any blood loss and the possible development of shock. You would also notify her physician of any increase in the size of the hematoma or changes in vital signs. Discomfort experienced by women after birth is often overlooked. By your thought processes and nursing actions, you have done much to alleviate her discomfort.

8. Two key nursing assessments that would lead you to suspect subinvolution are failure of the uterus to decrease in size at the expected rate and prolongation of lochia rubra or return of lochia rubra after the first several days of the postpartal period. Breastfeeding assists in involution, as you know, but you should not rule out the possibility of subinvolution in breastfeeding mothers if these signs exist.

9. Administer oral Methergine and antibiotics as ordered; encourage increase in fluid intake and a diet high in iron and multivitamins; do pad counts or weigh peri-pads (1g = 1 mL).

10. d   11. b   12. d

13. See text, pp. 1166–1167.

14. Evaluative outcome findings would include the following: exhibits signs of wound healing, such as decreased drainage, swelling, or redness of tissues; has a normal temperature; demonstrates increased tolerance for ambulation; understands treatment regimen, self-care, preventive measures, and implications for the care of her newborn.

Your evaluative outcome criteria may differ from these but should address some of these aspects.

15. Instruct the mother to take the entire course of prescribed antibiotics; foster rest; instruct her to avoid use of tampons or douches or having intercourse until she is told she can resume these activities; schedule follow-up visit; encourage increased fluid intake and diet high in protein and vitamin C.

16. Jeanne McGuire is at risk for overdistention of her bladder. Her risk factors included regional anesthesia and birth of twins (overdistention of the uterus). In addition, your physical findings that would support your response of "yes" are the following: the uterus is above the umbilicus and displaced to the right (by the distended bladder), and there is an increase in vaginal bleeding because the uterus cannot contract adequately.

Initial therapy is directed toward assisting her to empty her bladder: for example, pouring warm water over the perineum; providing pain medication as needed before her attempt to void; and applying ice packs to the perineum immediately postpartum to minimize edema, which can interfere with voiding. If these measures do not assist Jeanne to void, then catheterization may be done.

17. Answers may include the following: teach prevention by encouraging client to increase fluid intake, void after intercourse, and use cotton crotch underwear; and teach proper perineal hygiene.

18. Traumatized tissue: fissured or cracked nipples; overdistention: milk stasis.

19. Answers may include fever, chills, malaise, tachycardia, headache, flulike symptoms, and warm, reddened, painful areas.

20. Analgesics for discomfort, antibiotics, bed rest, increased fluid intake, supportive bra, frequent feeding of baby.

21. Answers may include increased amounts of clotting factors; presence of normal postpartal thrombocytosis; release of thromboplastin substances from tissues of decidua, placenta, and fetal membranes; and increased amounts of fibrinolysis inhibitors.

22. See text p. 1177, Table 38–7.

23. a   24. b   25. a   26. c   27. b   28. c

29. b   30. a   31. c

32. protamine sulfate

33. b

34. See text, pp. 1180–1183. Nursing Care Plan: The Woman with Thromboembolic Disease

35. See text, pp. 1183–1184.